Fred's Not Here

*Living with Alzheimer Disease
Takes Courage*

Lynn Smith

Previous books by Lynn Smith
Whitehorn Publishing

Gender or Giftedness: a challenge to rethink the basis for leadership in the faith community
first edition 2000; reprint 2009

Mentoring: Leaving a Legacy 2009

National Library of Canada Cataloguing in Publication

Smith, Lynn

Fred's Not Here: Living with Alzheimer Disease takes Courage/Lynn Smith

ISBN 978-0-9810460-2-0

Copyright © 2014 Lynn Smith

To order: Search online or contact Lynn Smith lynn@smithhouse.ca

Picture of Fred's Not Here Restaurant, Toronto ON Canada - used with permission

Table of Contents

DEDICATION		1
PREFACE		2
WHERE'S FRED?		3
Section I The Need for Courage		7
A.	Living with Fear	7
B.	Courage Givers	11
C.	Caregivers also Live with Fear	12
D.	Courage for the Caregivers	13
Section 2 My Story		15
A.	The Move to Toronto	16
	1. Trauma	16
	2. Settling In	19
	3. Ongoing Confusion	30
	4. New Perspective	34
	5. Surgery Anticipated	34
	6. Misspent Energy	35
	7. Missed Clues	38
	8. Added Assistance	46
B.	The Nursing Home	55
	1. Another Trauma	55
	2. The Difficult Decisions Continue	59
	3. Surgery and Unexpected Consequences	60
	4. Where's Fred?	64
	5. The Final Journey Home	67
C.	Eulogy for Mom	68

Section 3 Lessons Learned 73

    A.   Early Preparation 73

        1.   Pay attention to early signs 73
        2.   Find a doctor who will listen to your concerns 74
        3.   Recognize the uniqueness of dementia 74
        4.   Invest in an identification bracelet 74
        5.   Understand that dementia is unpredictable 74
        6.   Access all the resources you can 75

    B.   Living as the Caregiver 76

        1.   Put an alarm on the door before you need it 76
        2.   Enjoy the humorous in the midst of the difficulties 76
        3.   Stop to think who you are doing something for 76
        4.   Anticipate sudden uncharacteristic behaviours 77
        5.   Rethink the consequences of any surgery 77
        6.   Enter into their world 78
        7.   Recognize that loss of memory means the loss of a sense of time 78

    C.   Caring for Yourself 79

        1.   Remember that forgetting things is not the same as dementia 79
        2.   Be prepared to lose the person piece by piece 79
        3.   Find support for yourself as well as the one you care for 80
        4.   Learn how to grieve well 81
        5.   Know that encouragement requires truth and compassion 81
        6.   Take time to be still with God 83

POSTSCRIPT - 2014 85

APPENDIX 87

ABOUT THE AUTHOR 97

This is just a note to advise you that
Fred did not come to his bed last night
---

1 no excuse

2 no note

3 just absent without cause?

I am worried (naturally) and sleepy
What should I do or what can I do -
he may have been struck by someone!

Fred has gone somewhere --I am lost and alone, next door.
mom A

> Please find Fred and tell him to come and "take me home" please - I am lost. The only place I know is our old home and I can't find it. I am really lost - Fred will understand
> (I hope)

> Dear Lynn,
> I feel lost. Where am I and what do I do now? It is terrible to feel this way. Where am I and how do I get home? Please try to understand.
> I love you. MFA

Dedication

I dedicate this to my mother who lived the last years of her life in the memory-world of her childhood and to God who was present to her in those memories just as surely as he is present to me today. There is a timelessness in eternity that is perhaps most real to those who cannot remember the present.

I also dedicate this to our eldest grandchild, Alicia, who had a special relationship with her great-grandmother. I still have the necklace she made for her Great-grandma to wear in heaven, and the memory of her stroking Mom's cheek as she lay in bed during the last days and saying, "I just love her!" is a picture I will always cherish.

I want to express my profound gratitude to caregiver Marcia who gave Mom such loving care, Linda who by "living in" provided much needed freedom for us in the evenings, friend Margaret who shared Mom's love of art and enriched her life with trips to art galleries and visits with friends for afternoon tea, sister Gayle and brother John whose unquestioning support sustained me, my husband Roger who uncomplainingly made room for his mother-in-law in his heart and home, and all those too numerous to mention who chose to see Mom with eyes of kindness and hearts of grace when it would have been so easy to say, "She won't remember me so there's no point in speaking to her!"

And finally, I dedicate this to the countless caregivers who come alongside those who have lost their way in the fog of confusion. You are the unsung heroes. May God give you strength and courage and wisdom – and a supportive community.

Preface

Caring for someone with dementia is in some ways like having a child – there is no real preparation for it and each experience is unique; however, there are enough similarities that someone else's experience can perhaps be helpful.

I know it would have been encouraging for me to have someone to talk to who understood the journey from the caregiver's perspective: the gradual loss, the inconsistencies, the pain of making difficult decisions, the sense of failure at coming to the end of your ability to continue, the utter exhaustion, the fear of making poor decisions and the reality of having to make them.

Much has changed in the years since I cared for Mom. There are various medications available now. Government support systems have made it easier to keep someone in your home. Medical staff are more familiar with the characteristics of dementia.

So why write my story now?

I see around me friends and loved ones who are beginning the caregiving journey and my deep desire is to assist them in that journey by sharing some things I learned – things I wish I had known earlier in my own care-giving role. My journal reveals how much energy I expended trying to keep Mom sorted out – trying to talk with her as if she could remember, trying to pull her back to reality. I learned the hard way. Others will, too, of course. But perhaps some of my "lessons learned" will ease the way.

If what I learned can spare someone else even a small amount of the pain that I experienced in losing my mother inch by inch and agonizing over how to care for her in the process without diminishing her as a person and ensuring that her dignity was honoured, then this book will have fulfilled its purpose.

Where's Fred?

As Mom looked around the room, we anticipated her familiar question, "Where's Fred?"

Fred was her anchor, although even if he had been in the room, she wouldn't have recognized the old man that he had become. She was looking for the man she had married almost 60 years ago although even

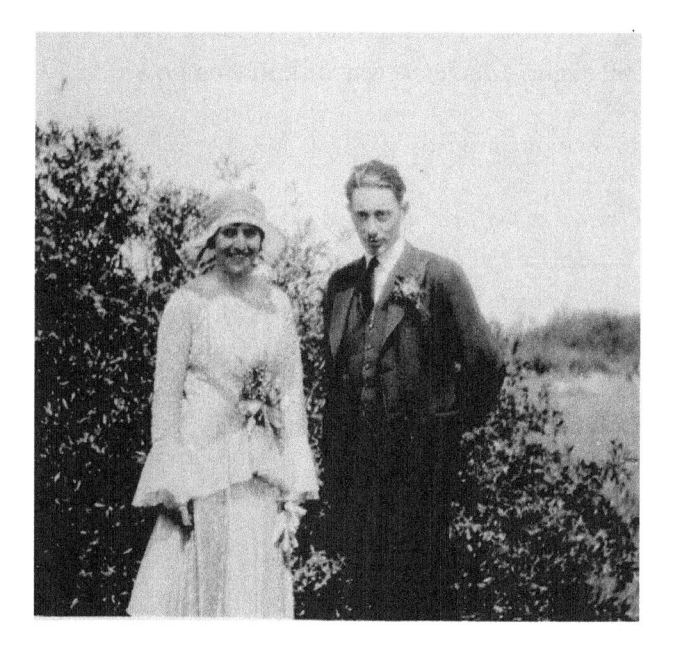

that memory was sometimes elusive as this note reveals.

> Lynn - Today
> A long time ago it seems that I got married - please come in to tell me about it - I feel lost again about certain events - Mom A

And we gave her our familiar response, "Fred's not here." It might be "Fred's not here tonight, or this time, or yet," and it seemed to settle her – for a few minutes at least.

The other questions she grappled with were not quite so easily answered:

> *Where is God in all of this? What have I done wrong to deserve this? Why?*

Her theology was so distorted. Was she reverting to her childhood understanding of God as a punishing God or had she never really worked that through? I have no way of knowing now.

And I had my own questions:

> *Is God limited by our final words? by our confusion? If he is merciful enough to cover the sins of his children, is he not also merciful enough to cover their confusion, their lack of understanding, the breakdown of their minds?*

Eventually, I realized that God was asking me to trust his character. I simply had to surrender my mother to the loving mercy of an all-knowing, wise God who is bigger than anything this world can bring our way.

Understanding the magnitude of God's grace and mercy came through the struggle of trying to make sense of what is senseless and accepting the impossibility of succeeding. I had to believe that God understood her heart and would help me to as well. Separating her heart and her spirit from her confused mind helped me to be able to care for her myself and also to draw others into the circle of care-giving. This became my ministry.

Ministry to me is meeting someone at their point of need. Some ministry needs are sudden, short-term, and usually obvious in nature. Others are ongoing, gradually wearing a person down, less identifiable although not less traumatic. That's the reality of being a caregiver.

Consequently, caregivers need to have a variety of support people in their lives – and it's especially helpful to have someone who has walked the journey before them.

One of the most important lessons I eventually learned was to at least attempt to see the world through her eyes. Mom helped me do that through the multitude of notes she wrote. I have interspersed this book with a sampling of those poignant notes that give a glimpse into her jumbled and fearful world.

Mom's notes – some scanned and others typed because they were in pencil or red ink which wouldn't scan well – are shown in the boxes throughout and a few more added in the appendix. They are just a sampling of the hundreds of notes I have kept. Rereading them has been heart wrenching as I heard and felt once again my mother's deep anguish at not knowing where she was or how to get home and especially thinking she had been abandoned by her husband and family.

Recently I have come to realize the value of my mother's ability to express her ongoing confusion and sense of abandonment. No doubt the feelings are common to those with dementia but unless they can express themselves, caregivers miss the intensity of their "lostness." Mom's messages, then, become her gift to those who share the same affliction by helping their caregivers understand a little better how frightening it is to not know where you are, how you got there or how you can get home again.

Section I is really an illustration of why it takes courage to live with Alzheimer Disease – whether you are the person with dementia or the caregiver.

Section II is my story of being the caregiver told through the sporadic writing of journals and a few letters to keep my father and siblings informed, along with some illustrations of how consistently confusing and progressively narrowing the world is for someone with dementia.

In order to reveal with raw honesty my struggles, mistakes and consequent insights, I have chosen to not edit my journals.

Section III is a collation of the various lessons learned through my experience. You may choose to read through my journal to see the progress and note the lessons learned throughout or simply skip to the last section for the "lessons" and then if you need further background, you can go back to the journal entry that gives more detail.

One lesson I'll mention here is that it's important to seek out resources as soon as you suspect dementia because once you are in a care-giving role, you will have neither the time nor the energy to attend seminars or check out resources. That's when you ask others to do the research for you.

Section I The Need for Courage

A. Living with Fear

There is nothing about my mother that would indicate the reality that she faces almost constant fear. She looks bright, but she lives with the thief that is gradually and relentlessly robbing her of her memory which provides the link with the past, an understanding of the present and hope for the future.

> Dear Lynn —
> Why am I here?
> Where should I be?
> I need to go home but where is home?
> Please tell me all I need to know, please help.
> Mom. J.G.

Picture with me a woman who has been a school teacher, an artist, a friend. Someone who has had an interest in everything, but most keenly in her family – her children and grandchildren. Someone who lived through the depression on the prairies. Someone who had a faith in God that survived marriage to a declared agnostic. Someone who, when her husband went into the Air Force, left the city with three small children to teach ten grades in a small country school house, and who not too many years later set out on her own with two daughters on the train to make the move from Saskatchewan to British Columbia (leaving her husband and son to sell the house and follow later) because she needed to get there in time to start the fall school term as the new teacher. A woman of courage, strength, and creativity.

Now picture with me that same woman lost, bewildered, feeling abandoned by everyone she gave her life to, wondering how she could end up without any of her family; wondering how she got where she is and how she can ever find her way home; wondering why God is punishing her. What has she ever done to deserve this?

Is it Alzheimer Disease? It doesn't really matter what label it gets, the reality is that dementia is difficult – difficult for the person who has it and difficult for the family members who care.

Most people don't recognize the look of confusion and fear behind the pleasant smile: fear that she will say something weird and embarrass herself or someone else; fear that she will be thought crazy and be put away; fear of being lost in this bewildering world - drifting without any anchor except the physical presence of the person beside her with no memories to link the present to the past; experiencing the emotions of guilt when she thinks she must have left her husband and family, alternating with the hurt of rejection when she thinks they must have left her; and asking herself over and over again, won't I ever get my memory back again? Why isn't there any cure? Why would God let this happen to me?

Meet my mother – she could be sitting next to you in church.

She has been married for almost 60 years and now she is separated from her husband – a sad and confusing experience. Her thoughts race in confusion:

Have I done something I ought not to have done – why did I leave him? Or did he leave me? I must figure out some way to get to him, or at least to explain this strange circumstance – but I can't figure it out. What's wrong with me? It's just so muddled. The hymns - they're so familiar – so why am I confused? Where is everyone I've known? Where do I live? I must find my way back home? Home – ah yes –

and her mind settles on the only home she can remember with any clarity – that wonderful place where she was once young and free and happy – the farm home of her childhood. Why did she ever leave the farm, she wonders.

Once again she becomes the free spirit she once was. The young girl who dreamed of being a teacher who loved her pupils and felt a sense of usefulness as she poured herself into their lives. The young woman who developed a tenacity for facing hardship such as only those who pioneered on the harsh and cold prairies ever did. The young mother who coped through the depression and the bleak years which followed for those who lost their jobs, by going back to the farm, feeding farm-hands, making over old clothes, planting gardens and living the life that teaching and marriage to a banker had promised to rescue her from. She became in her day-dreaming the woman she recognized as capable, independent, competent, contributing to this world her energies and her creativity…..

but…what's this – we're all standing up and so, without warning, that image fades and she looks around her in bewilderment. Where has she gone – this person? It feels like me – but it cannot be for I do not know how I even got here. This person sitting next to me – she says she is my daughter – but when did she grow up. Who raised her? She's so kind to me and I can trust her somehow – I just know I can – so I'll have to ask her to help me figure this all out.

The hymns again – they really are familiar – but so little else is – I wonder why?

This is my mother, Mary Frances. But she could be one of many others in your community.

Her loss of memory means the loss of everything in the past that has given meaning to her life. It also means the loss of any sense of security – nothing is familiar so everything is always changing.

> *I must remember. I do hope to remember so many experiences of long ago, in our childhood days –*
>
> *I hope John & Ruth will come to pick me up. –*
>
> *Am I at home now?*
>
> *Please Talk –*
>
> *get Fred to come if he is able.*

Imagine waking up every morning in an environment you don't recognize – not knowing where you are or how you got there. That's enough fear for anyone.

But there's an even deeper fear – the loss of purpose and identity. There is no connectedness to people in the present or to achievement in the past. Meaning, security and purpose – spell IDENTITY!! If you lose all three, you lose a sense of who you are.

This woman needs to be encouraged. She needs courage to trust when there is no memory, courage to face a new world almost every day for there is often only a vague sense of familiarity about her surroundings, courage to accept the unacceptable, courage to find the funny side of things – to laugh at herself and circumstances to ease the torment and frustration, courage to believe that God is in control of what feels so out of control.

B. Courage Givers

> Am I lost? Where should I go? I thought someone would help me by now? <u>Lynn</u> – why – (get the police if worried) <u>Please</u> <u>help</u> – I <u>need</u> <u>your</u> <u>help</u> now to know what, why, and where I should go= Please explain "<u>to help</u> – why, where and when (I need to know) so do you – Love Mom F.
>
> I don't want to get sick and just now I feel it – Where is Fred, why am I lost? and alone? (Please explain) if Fred is happy, then I will not worry – but let me <u>know</u> Mom A.
>
> Fred will have to tell me <u>what,</u> and <u>why</u> and tell me what to expect and do.

How do you give courage to one who is so lost?

There are a multitude of small ways.

In light of her disconnectedness, it is encouraging when she is remembered and touched and hugged and fussed over. She feels welcomed and her response is that this must be where she belongs because people remember HER even when she can't remember them.

Not everyone knows how desperately she needs to feel that she belongs, but one who understood ministered to her deepest need one Sunday when she lost sight of me and confided in the person next to her that she was lost. The response was a warm and loving, "Oh no, you're not lost - you've been FOUND!"

She is affirmed by those who enjoy her wit and gentle nature, who recognize and call forth her creativity, who see her as a person and who can help her recall her past achievements and see value in those. These are people who look for the source of her identity that is so fleeting for her.

She is also affirmed by those who allow her the freedom to ask the bewildering questions, even when they may have just answered them a dozen times. One dear man pushes his way through whoever is blocking his path until he gets close enough to take her hand in both of his and give her a warm handshake and big smile. His English is limited and so he says very little or nothing at all – but she feels welcomed. He is not afraid of her disability – and recognizes her need. He has courage and he encourages – although he would not even realize that he has "ministered" to anyone.

These are the angels unaware.

C. Caregivers also Live with Fear

Those who care for the memory-impaired loved ones have a different set of fears. Caregivers are reluctant to let anyone know they are having difficulty coping because at the very least it feels like complaining – if not outright betrayal. The onset is so subtle and gradual that it's easy to dismiss until something drastic happens. After all, don't we all forget things? Care-givers fear not doing the right thing; they fear belittling their partner or parent; they fear what will happen if the person gets lost; they fear driving with them and fear having to take away their license; they fear leaving them alone and fear having someone stay with them to give them a break; they fear the future in a different way from the one with dementia. The one with dementia is confused in the present; for the caregiver, the present may be manageable, at least for the moment, but the future is frightening. They, too, need encouragement.

D. Courage for the Caregivers

Encouragement for caregivers comes from having a few people around them who will:

- enter into the pain with them without thinking they have to take it away
- give time and opportunity to process new information
- allow space for healing
- ask how they're feeling rather than assuming
- let them talk – and really LISTEN!
- acknowledge the reality, and the emotions
- focus on them and their current needs rather than themselves
- alleviate responsibilities – do something FOR them
- offer what they are able to give – be specific and creative

The gifts of compassion that made the journey a little less stressful for me included having someone to give me a few hours respite from the constant questions by taking Mom for a drive or visiting her at home; going with me to check out nursing homes when that time came; providing around-the-clock watchcare for Mom after her eye surgery to keep her from removing the bandage.

These may have seemed like small things to the people offering them but they made a significant difference to me.

Section 2 My Story

Places referred to in the journal entries:

- Toronto, Ontario – where I live
- Clearbrook, BC – where my parents lived
- Salem, Oregon – where my aunt Grace lived
- The farm – where Mom grew up near Watrous, Saskatchewan

Identity of the people mentioned (listed alphabetically):

- Alicia – my granddaughter – son Malcolm's daughter
- Brad – Gayle's son (Cindy –his wife)
- Brenda – Gayle's daughter (Gord – her husband)
- Darrell – my son
- Don and Jessie – Grace's son (my cousin) and his wife
- Elda and Ken – my cousin and her husband
- Fred – my Father
- Gayle and Gerry – my sister and her husband
- George Sager – long-time friend of Fred's who introduced him to Mom
- Grace – my mother's sister
- John and Ruth – my brother and his wife
- Julie and Dave – my daughter and her husband
- Karen – daughter of friends
- Ken and Luella – Karen's parents and long-time friends
- Linda – seminary student who came to live with us
- Little John – my brother's grandson
- Malcolm and Miriam – my son and his wife
- Marcia – the caregiver we hired to be with Mom on weekdays
- Mary Frances – my Mother
- Maybelle – Mom's sister who died many years before Mom
- Roger – my husband
- Roy and Win – Mom's brother and his wife

A. The Move to Toronto

1. Trauma

There are a number of events that remain starkly embedded in my memory; however, the reasons behind those events are only recorded because I periodically journalled my thoughts, as I shared Mom's journey.

One of the most traumatic events was bringing my mother to live with us in Toronto.

My father, at age 90, had burned out. None of the family lived close enough to give him the support he would need to continue coping with Mom, whose behavior had become erratic and accusatory. He had tried having her stay occasionally in a respite care home for a break but she phoned him repeatedly to come and get her.

September 1988

Dad called and for the first time, I think, I've really been able to say that separating them would be better than the way things are now. I think I've not wanted to admit to that before because I thought that would be so hard on Mom. But Mom was ready to pack up and leave then and there!! I've heard about a place in White Rock and have called, but the section that would suit their needs best hasn't been built yet.

I've even wondered about bringing Mom back here. She says every once in a while now that she wants to go home and it's always back to the farm. She sometimes asks Dad where she's to sleep – who she's to sleep with – why they're staying there, when they can go home again, etc., etc., so if she does that here, it wouldn't be much different, and would give Dad a break.

October 19, 1988

Well, it looks as if that's what I'm going to do. As a family, we made the decision that the best place for Mom was in our home in Toronto. Julie and I will fly out in December, celebrate Dad's 90th birthday and then pack up Mom to bring her home. Dad won't come to live in Toronto, so he will sell their house and move to live near Gayle. I will need to find someone to come in on the days I work who will be a companion for Mom but who does enough around the house to make Mom think that she's here to work for me.

In some ways it's pretty scary to think of the change in lifestyle it will mean for us. At other times it's a relief to have made a decision. I know that I may not be able to keep her at home – that she may need to go into a home – but I will at least have the comfort of knowing that I gave it a try. If she were to go into a home in Clearbrook, she would be most unhappy because she'd see it as a rejection.

(*Postscript 2014* Little did I know that she would still see coming to Toronto as rejection – not just by Dad but by the whole family as she gradually lost her memory of who we are.)

December 23, 1988

Two weeks ago in Clearbrook we had a wonderful party for Dad and packed up all Mom's stuff. All of the family from out West were there. Beginning Thursday evening people continued to arrive until the dinner party Saturday night, and then the departures began Sunday morning which was really difficult because most of them had the experience of saying good-bye to Mom and for the first time, thinking that maybe they wouldn't see her again. We've always dealt with that every time we've gone out West – but for them, it was a first. Then we had to deal with Dad having nothing to say to Mom about leaving. He has never said much – but I found it hard to cope with this time. The memory of seeing Dad say goodbye to Mom who could not understand why she was going with me – and Fred wasn't – still brings tears. And we also had to deal with Mom not really understanding because no one else has had the courage to tell her she has Alzheimer disease and even if they had, she probably wouldn't have remembered. Dad hadn't even said she was going to live with me, but left it for me to do. I couldn't just up and leave with her without letting the people there know and so I arranged an open house as well as getting to the bank and the doctor and getting her some clothes and getting her hair done. It has been really hard on her to come at Christmas and many times I've wondered what in the world I was doing bringing her down here. Maybe it would have been better to let her be neglected where she was than to do something so traumatic. It's hard to know what is best for someone else.

Later reflection

That decision was hard, but it was just the first of a multitude that, because they were less traumatic than this major move, surprised me with how draining they were. I'm referring to those daily decisions about how to respond to someone who is your mother but has become a dependent child – someone who, unlike a child, is not growing and developing but deteriorating; who is inconsistent in her responses and abilities; who asks adult questions but cannot reason enough to struggle with answers; who needs constant reassurance because of her constant fear.

Those were the daily decisions that confronted me – how to respond to confusion and fear that never seemed to diminish. I found it to be more draining than I could have anticipated. And the move clearly confused her more than ever. This note indicates that she thought John and Gayle were her brother and sister instead of her children and that she had no idea she had left Clearbrook.

There is something wrong about the days and the time of the year, etc. I would like to phone my brother John Hoover, and sister Gayle Macaulay - Please try to contact them for me - I'm "Frances, Hoover" "Adcock" and I want to see my family, John, Hoover and Ruth, Gayle and Gerry Macaulay, Maybelle and family, PLEASE. I am living in a home in Clearbrook - Please try to find me. I need family.

2. Settling In

December 27, 1988

Mom has had a lot of difficulty settling in here at Christmas. It is the first time in 58 years that she has not been with Dad at Christmas and it is really hard for her to understand WHY!! And then when she does understand, she forgets – so we go over it again and again. I wish I had kept a diary of the last weeks – but I've been too busy living it to write anything down. However, things do seem to be much better now for her. One real blessing is that she can talk about her feelings and another is that she really likes Marcia. Hiring Marcia was one very positive decision. She has "adopted" Mom and they have a happy relationship.

The same themes keep coming up over and over again. It has been hard for her to give up her home. She still asks consistently,

> *What does Fred think about my being here? Why doesn't he come to see me? What does the rest of the family think? What a terrible way to end up! Where is my money? I need to pay you for being here! I need to be independent! Where is Fred? I need to go home tomorrow! How do I get there? Why am I here? When will I get my memory back? If I get it back will Fred take me back again? What can I do to fix this mess?*

Mom leaves notes for me – or for herself – or for someone – written on anything she can find: old envelopes, books, scrap paper, cards, note paper.

> Lynn, I am upstairs in a big room & double bed so if you get too tired come up & see me (awaken me)

Dear Fred,—
  I am so sorry to be alone and "sort of lost." This family are good to me but I do miss the rest, just hope they will come to visit.
  @ John & Ruth, Gayle & Jerry; Lynn is a regular visitor which we enjoy. Roger, her husband comes with Lynn.
  Please "let me" have a visit with my old friends. I miss them and feel sad, we left in to big a hurry. Love
                                    Frances
  I need advice and help.

  I need to go home and I need help to get there.
      Thanks & Love
          M. F. A

Gradually I'm beginning to see a shift. Mom now can hardly remember Clearbrook, although she recognizes pictures and knows they are of her home. She can't believe she hasn't been here for a long time. On the way home from Julie's on Christmas day, she said that she wanted to go home "tomorrow" – because she wanted to be back with "the family" but I laid out once again the various "options" – and she agreed that none of them was possible. So then she asked, "Why can't I live with you?" I told her she could and that we wanted her to, but that she didn't seem to want to, to which she replied, in tears, that it was too much to ask. She really sees herself as a burden, a nuisance, and wants to know what the rest of the family thinks about my being stuck with her!! And what are they doing to help me? No amount of reassurance has yet sunk in but hopefully in time it will. She's worried about getting worse and keeps asking if there isn't anything she can do to help her memory, or can't the doctors do anything.

I have needed the courage to tell her the truth about herself. There is a reason for her condition. It may not be pleasant or even acceptable – but it's understandable. It helps to cut through her guilt at being the way she is and where she is – at least for the moment.

As the questions are repeated, my answers tend to be variations on the following:

> Lynn Please take me home-- That is "take me to Fred's place (that is mine also)" I need to have someone to talk to, not to scold me as that seems to be all anyone _does_. Take me to my Dad's home up on the Hill.
> Please ---.F.A. _thanks_

> *Mom, you have Alzheimer's. No, you cannot do anything about it. No, you cannot live alone. No, you cannot go back and keep house for Dad. Your only other option to being here is to be in a nursing home. No, you are not stupid – you have a disease that makes you forget. No, you aren't a burden. And no, you haven't done anything wrong.*

And then countering the "no's" with some "yeses."

> *Yes, I am your daughter – all grown up. Yes, I know you. Yes, your family all love you. Yes, Fred is your husband and he is well and he knows you are here. Yes, God knows you are here with me. Yes, it is safe here. Yes, we want you here with us. Yes, you have enough money to last you as long as you live.*

I have also attempted to help her validate her fears and losses.

> *It must be scary to feel like you're lost. It must be hard to give up your own home. When you don't remember the family you must feel abandoned. Yes, it's hard to feel useless. You're not, you know – what would you like to do? You don't have to DO anything to be loved. You can lie in bed the rest of your life and DO NOTHING if you want – but you are still my mother – and that's what makes you important to me – not what you do.*

Facing her fears meant reassuring her frequently about the two things that worried her most: money and family. She needed to not be dependent financially, and she needed to be connected with family. So these messages, too, were frequently required.

> *You have money in the bank. Dad isn't taking your money. Your pension is coming directly to your bank. You can contribute to your room and board if you wish. You can take money out anytime you like. You have enough money to travel so you can visit the family.*

> *You can phone any of the family anytime. You can write to them anytime. Everyone is sad that you have to be here. Everyone is happy that you are here. Everyone knows that family is important to you.*

> *The family can visit you here. You can invite anyone at anytime. We have extra beds for visitors.*

Malcolm and Miriam have dropped Alicia in while they shopped with Julie and Dave. Mom is so thrilled to be holding her. When we were out West, Mom was so uncharacteristically sharp with little John (one more early indicator of her dementia) and I have to admit that I was concerned about how I'd deal with her around Alicia on a continuing basis so it has been a big relief to have her be so receptive to Alicia. Hopefully it will be a positive relationship for both of them.

(Postscript 2014 And it definitely was – for both of them!)

January 3, 1989

It gets pretty tedious – but Marcia is a real answer to prayer – she is just wonderful with Mom and Mom enjoys her. She takes her for walks, reads Mom's poetry to her, gets her to help fold the laundry and generally keeps her pretty well occupied without being bossy. This week people are back to their offices and I'm beginning to get somewhere with Rehab, Seniors assessment, etc.

Mom has started a letter to John and Ruth to say thanks for the track suit and the blue cotton dress – I doubt that it will get finished but I'll send it as is. I told her I was writing to them and did she wish to say anything - she said to say, "Hi and I love you both."

Mom has written to Gayle and Gerry. She was wearing the dressing gown they sent – loves it and has worn nothing else since!! And I put the drawer liners next to her on her desk. She must have asked me fifteen times what she was to do them and who sent them. Then I left her to write in the card she bought for them last week. (I took her shopping one day and she thought she was in Vancouver!) When I came back she had written a little in the card but mostly on the sheet of paper that was intended to be her check list. I decided it was better to just send it all the way it was. If I tried to get her to copy it over onto a separate sheet, they might never get it.

Marcia is going to help her put the liners into the drawer – she can't seem to comprehend what that box is and every time I tell her that Gayle and Gerry sent the dressing gown – she looks surprised and so delighted.

Mom's way of de-stressing was to write notes. I have a drawer full of her anxious ones. These are some happy ones, even if the facts are confused.

> Dear Everyone
>
> I have decided that the world is a lovely place to live in. I have lived all my life thinking that I have to do something to have value and I have worked hard all my life to always be doing doing doing. Now I am ready to sit back and enjoy just being who I am. I can do things because I want to do them, but I don't HAVE to do anything.
>
>   Love Grandma

Dear Family

This is the Day after the night before - I am all alone in "my" room which is a nice big room with a big double bed, and a "gold" cloth spread -- It also has a dresser, a "shif" a book case of books and a "big enough" closet for my 3 dresses and boots. I hope you can come and visit me here. It feels so much better since the Smith's bought it. I do hope everything turns out ok for the buyers -- and I do hope you will all be able to come to visit.

I am quite well and happy now that I do not have to move out. I will have to learn what Fred will do or go or plan next. I am going to go to bed now - (This last sentence wore me out) so will add more when I wake up tomorrow, I think and hope everything will be ok as it sounds too good to be real. Will add more tomorrow.

Goodnight -

This is tomorrow morning and a beautiful sunny one - I do need friends and a "reason" for everything -- Why am I here and alone -- I need someone to talk to not just to look at - Is this a hospital? or is it a home for the forgotten? Please be a friend and talk to me.

As ever, Frances.

It is so good and really wonderful to know I have such wonderful daughters — I hope they enjoy their families as I have mine. My sorrow is that I have not seen them enough.

I do want to see them again so will try, that is I must work on "the idea" of seeing them again, it may be more than I can manage but will try. When I take time to look & think about them I feel sad as I have been sort of boxed in so did not get around as I should have liked.

Will try harder now
love man A

Dad seemed to always have others to visit with except his family — and they understood to their sorrow.

This is Lynn's home and I live here with them — I don't have to leave and I feel safe and not alone.

---

also —

I need a box? of paints & some brushes — it would be a thank you parcel — maybe I should find my old ones

I must remember this — I like all of it.

Reach up as far as you can... and God will reach down the rest of the way.

Thank you —

> I will say Goodnight and happy dreams as I will be on my way as early as possible.
>
> So have a Happy New Year and many more
>
> Love Gram

January 13, 1989

I feel as if we had a real break-through today. Mom cried about Dad, saying that she felt so sorry for him being all alone with no one to care for him. She said that she likes it so much here that she feels she is just being selfish. That Dad has come to the time of life when he should be thinking about things at a deeper level and that she hasn't tried hard enough to talk to him – that she should do something.

> Just me
> I don't want to just sit, nor to fiddle my life away, what is left of it is precious. I need to organize the rest of my days. I want to talk to John - he has a good head and will understand and realize what is necessary for me to do "yet" so please help.
> Please let me go to visit with him and talk things over. But first would like to visit with the family here (those close) as well as far away, Mom A

Uselessness is a recurring theme and we have had so many conversations about it that I began to get underneath her thinking patterns by asking what she thought God wanted her to do with her life. Her answer was that she should do her best, no matter what. That's a standard answer and is so subtle in its lie that it's hard to talk against. But I tried by asking her what would happen if she didn't do her best. She made fun of it by jesting that maybe she'd be sent to the devil. The sad part is that I think there's some uncertainty under that jest. So I pressed her for an answer. If going to be with God depends on our doing our best – then no one will ever succeed because no one ever does their best ALL the time. Scripture in fact teaches quite the reverse – that Jesus invites the broken and the sinner and the outcast to come – it is in the act of coming that we are cleansed and made welcome and accepted – not in the process of trying to make ourselves acceptable. That is something that we cannot do.

We went on to talk about her need to be useful and I pointed out that our usefulness to God is not in being a good teacher or mother or whatever – that our purpose on earth is to reflect Christ to the world – and that means that her usefulness is no less today than it was when she was an active teacher many years ago. Her sphere of influence has changed but not her usefulness. In fact, in many ways it has increased because she now has more time to devote to "talking to God" about all her family. Last night we drew a tree – she was the trunk and John, Gayle and I were the three main branches – with the grandchildren branching off them and then the great-grandchildren. The root represented her ancestors giving her their heritage. We talked about the need for her to recognize that she had not come to a "gap" in her life like she felt, but that she could now rest peacefully in the shade of her offspring – recognizing that she has given them life and now she can relax and just enjoy her "life-giving" and nurturing action of the past.

Today, I built on that image by suggesting that she had given physical life to all those people, now, perhaps God was calling her to be the channel for them to have spiritual life – that by spending her time in prayer for all her family she could have the most useful period of her life.

Several years ago when Mom visited and I took her to my Bible study, she asked the ladies to pray over her. She had a vision of herself in the center of a huge room that looked like the entrance to a palace. She seemed to want to go in but a voice told her that she was not to enter yet – that she was to go back because there was something yet that she had to do. She has never known what that was – although she seems to remember the event. Today, I told her that this is what I thought God was asking of her – to reflect Him to her family and to be that channel of his blessing to each one. She had such a sense of peace come over her and said she felt so calm – the first time for so long – almost as if a new spirit had come upon her.

Then after supper, she was sitting in her room when I went up to tell her we were going for a walk and she said she was so contented – this was such a peaceful house – why was that? She said that if she went home she would be agitated again. I said that the Peace of God was in our home. She misunderstood at first, thinking I meant her old home and cried saying, "I thought you meant in my home and I'd missed it!" We talked about how God's Spirit brings a spiritual unity that is deeper than the emotional one and I think for the first time that I understand the nature of her feeling of rejection by the family. When she can't remember the emotional connection, she feels its absence as rejection. I told her the family have not rejected her but here she has a spiritual unity that brings peace. I hope the peace lasts.

> Lynn is teaching - Roger is at work -- They have a maid so I'm just sitting and feeling sadder by the minute. I have a husband but where? and why - What is he doing about our home life? I need to know because it is part of living a normal life.

January 14, 1989

Our lives basically center around Mom these days, with a visit now and then from Alicia!! Last night Mom said again that she liked it so much here that she felt selfish.

January 20, 1989

Marcia is a miracle worker...Mom is painting! Last week she said that she was afraid to paint – afraid that she couldn't do it anymore. I asked her what would happen if she tried it and found she couldn't remember what to do. She said that people would laugh at her so I asked who she thought would laugh and her immediate response was, "No one in this house!" So I suggested she try and if she couldn't then no one would ever need to know, but if she could still paint, then we could tell people. I have no way of knowing what she processes and what she doesn't, but Marcia has persevered and she started on Wednesday and has done some each day.

Last night she said that she thought she should go home but that she didn't really want to – she was afraid to. She didn't think she could keep house anymore and besides there were people here to talk to. "My time is short now and I want to talk to people. I guess it bothered Fred that I wanted to talk. I'd be lonely at home."

3. Ongoing Confusion

January 22, 1989

I have had difficulty figuring out why Mom keeps talking about going home to the family – why not just going home to Fred? That is certainly there. She's constantly worrying about where Fred is and who's looking after him. The fact that he's at Gayle's is alternately "okay" because "*Gayle was always his favorite*" and "not okay" because he "*ought to have taken me, too,*" and couldn't she just go and why doesn't he come to get her! I can't seem to get her to hold onto the fact that we are family too. Well, yesterday it became clear that "family" was her family of origin – not any of us!! We were sitting at the table having breakfast and she said she wanted to go home to her family. I asked her who she was thinking of when she talked about family. She said, "Well, let me see – who is there? Well, there's Grace – she's married – probably her third or fourth husband!" I interjected that Grace was now a widow and living alone – that Arlie had died – maybe six or so years ago and her response was,

"How do you know all this?" I told her that I kept up with all the family and always had. She rephrased her question then, which was a revelation, "But why are you interested in all my family?" The ensuing conversation went something like this:

> *"I'm interested because I'm part of the family."*
> *"You are?"*
> *"Yes, I'm your daughter."*
> *"Well, why have you kept that from me for so long? Why haven't you told me?"*
> *"I have, Mom, but you've forgotten. If you don't think of me as your daughter, who am I?"*
> *"You're a very nice lady who has taken in an old lady and given me a home."*
> *"You mean like a stranger?"*
> *"Oh, no, you're not a stranger."*
> *"Then, how am I connected to you?"*
> *"Well, it seems that you came into my life as a little girl, and I've kept track of you all these years."*
> *"I did! And you did! Because I am your daughter and you raised me."*
> *"Well, then, who's your father?"*

I joked with her about that – saying that if she didn't know who my Father was, what kind of past did she have!! I've done that before and she's laughed with me but this time she was really serious and repeated it so I told her, "Fred."

> *"Fred is your father!!! How could he be — he's got such a queer nature."*
> *"If he had such a queer nature, how come you married him?"*
> *"I suppose I was in love with him."*
> Then I told her Julie was arriving any minute and asked if she knew who Julie was.
> *"Yes."*
> *"Do you know she's your grand-daughter?"*
> *"Vaguely."*
> *"Do you know she's my daughter?"*
> *"How could that be? "*

Just then Julie arrived, greeted her and then went to make herself some coffee. Mom was so dumbfounded that she knew her way around the kitchen.

"It looks like you've been here before. How do you know where everything is and I don't."
"Well, I used to live here, Grandma."
"You're the one who sent me to the hospital?" (pointing to me)
"Yezz ma'am. I sure did. And do you remember that I started to come backwards and they had to push me back in and turn me around."
"Where was I?"
"In lots of pain, most likely!!"
"And who is she?" (pointing to Julie)
"She's the one who sent me to the hospital. She's my daughter and I'm your daughter!!"
"Isn't that wonderful – but why haven't I known this? Where have I been? What's wrong with me?"

February 1989

Mom is forever packing her suitcase. It's so heavy I can hardly lift it and yet she can get it downstairs ready to "go home" at a moment's notice!! I've tried to convince her to let me put it away but it seems to be her security and she wants it under her bed.

> John came to visit today - It was good to see him again and looking so well.

Darrell is taking Mom out to Hamilton on Saturday to spend the day with Julie. She seems much less agitated now than she was for a while. She still thinks she's visiting and gets concerned about how and when she's going home – more "how" than "when" it seems now. She is always disoriented when we come back home after I have taken her anywhere. Some days she still hunts for her suitcase, but doesn't usually pack it anymore. Sometimes she'll be content if I tell her where it is and that she can always get it when it's needed. If anyone asks her where she lives, it's still Clearbrook, and she still pines for Fred – feeling sorry that he's all alone and thinking she should go to be with him, and alternately feeling angry that he has pushed her out.

Dad sent the real-estate forms and she signed them without any hesitation – saying afterward, "It makes me sad." I queried, "Because it's the end of an era?" Her response was, "It makes the difference between having a house and NOT having a house." That is a big issue for her. It has always been important for her to have her own home.

> Where should I be now? At Home - but where is home? I'd love it if I could find it, or really see it. All I want is to have a home, to be in a home, one I can call my own. Why can I not have one?
> I feel I must go away? My dad's hope is to find a resting place - I need a real home - my own to build up and make it a home.
> What are my troubles and why? I need to know what I can do.
> Love Frances
> I need my parents and the law and you-
> Love M.F.A

4. New Perspective

March 1989

We had such a wonderful time at Auntie Grace's Birthday and with Don and Jessie. It was a wonderful break for me to have no responsibility for a while. I just relaxed and gained some perspective on the situation with Mom. I had been too enmeshed in daily living to have time to sit back and reflect on what was happening – or to even comprehend the reality of it all. When I came home, it was with the realization that this was not something that was going to go away – that Mom wasn't going to "get over it" and be herself again. That was hard, but necessary.

> Lesson Learned: Caring for someone with dementia is very different from caring for someone who is eventually getting better, or someone with physical disabilities, or for a child who is developing. It's in a totally different category.

5. Surgery Anticipated

April 20, 1989

Have just returned from a visit to Princess Margaret Hospital – the first for me – to have an ultra sound done on Mom's left eye. The cataract is so thick that the Dr. couldn't see through it so wanted a picture to help decide the appropriateness of cataract surgery. He said that there was no point in putting her through surgery to remove the cataract, if, when it was done, she still couldn't see due to damage on the back of the eye. He was concerned because she sees only the left half of things with her left eye – possibly the result of a stroke – and a solid line appears broken which could indicate retina damage. However, everything looks good and we'll go ahead with the plans to have surgery sometime during the summer. I have been impressed by his thoroughness and his kindness and patience in dealing with Mom. His first step was to give me a prescription for a new lens for her good right eye, saying, "Let's give her the very best vision she can possibly have in that eye, then we'll work on the other eye."

Everything I've heard and seen makes me more and more angry with the kind of medical attention Mom and Dad were getting in Clearbrook.

> Lesson Learned: Find a doctor who will listen to you if you suspect dementia. I had gone with Mom to her doctor in Clearbrook who refused to listen to my concerns. He would ask Mom if she was forgetting things or if she had any dizzy spells recently. Of course she said, "No!" She wouldn't have remembered if she had. The doctor then inferred that I was an interfering daughter flying in from Toronto thinking that I knew more than he did.
>
> "Your mother is just fine. She should know!!" was his response to my concerns.
>
> Fortunately doctors are wiser today about dementia. They recognize that the family does know more than they do about changes in behaviour.

6. Misspent Energy

April 29, 1989

I've just had a session with Mom. We did up the supper dishes and she went in to watch TV. I sat with her for a while and then left to study for my exam. When I returned half an hour or so later, she was still in the big chair and Roger was with her watching TV. She said, "Oh you've come back, where did the rest of the girls go?" I tried to figure out what she was referring to and she got upset. She said she'd been left alone all afternoon in the chair deserted by everyone. What did she do? When I said there hadn't been anyone here today but us and told her what she'd done all evening, she wanted to know where Fred was, why didn't he come for her. Where was she to sleep tonight? Why was she here? Where had all her family gone? I should get the police to get after Fred to make him take his responsibility. Where was John – he would take her in and I said gently, "No, he wouldn't. He couldn't. He doesn't live at home half the time – he's living all across Canada with the pipe line and there's no way you could live with him, so you're stuck with us." She cried and said it's not me that's stuck with you it's you that's stuck with me." I said, "Don't talk that nonsense!" She cried and said she didn't want to live and I got cross with her. I told her to stop talking like that - that she was my mother and that she was the grandmother of my children and they needed her and wanted her. She cried, "Don't get cross with me." and I said, "Yes, I will – I want you to hear me!" Her response was, "Well, if that's the way I feel, why shouldn't I say it. It's awful when you've lived with someone and had children with them and then they throw you out like an old rag." I realized that she was right to express her feelings and because Fred doesn't want to live with her she thinks that she's pretty awful – so no one would want to. She said that she hopes none of the men follow his example. And then laughed and said she should write that down and send it to him.

> Lesson Learned: It's better to listen to feelings rather than words.

May 23, 1989

I am disappointed that Dad won't come here, but feel that I cannot persuade him to because I am not sure how quickly Mom's condition will deteriorate. There are times when she doesn't know that Fred is her husband although she always remembers "Fred". She always knows me, too, and all the rest of the family but she can't always remember the connection we have to her or to each other. Sometimes I'm her sister, sometimes her daughter, and sometimes that nice lady who has given her a place to live. She also cannot retain the fact that she is in Toronto and that the rest of the family is out west. She can't figure out why Fred doesn't come home, or come to pick her up, or why he left. Her confusion is a real problem to her because she knows she's confused and feels lost all the time. We are blessed with Marcia who comes in to look after her.

Sometimes we feel as though we are basically just coping, although we are always very much aware of God's goodness and the loving care of His people.

Mom is not good about going to bed at a regular time. One night she wrote this and left it by my door. It's quite revealing about her relationship with her father.

> Dear Fred,
>
> Today is Sunday afternoon and Lynn and I are having a talk. I am having difficulty remembering a lot of things and it really bothers me. I am sure it must have bothered you too. It sure bugs me. The things that are important to me - and important to everyone else - are so vague to me - I just don't understand.
>
> I don't know how to figure it out. I don't know how to handle it myself. Surely there must be someone, somewhere who can help.
>
> I remember the church this morning. I remember Lynn. But so many things are like dreams that fade away.
>
> I really miss you and wish you were here. I really like it here Everything is so peaceful here. I feel selfish being here when I worry about who's looking after you. After so many years together it seems so sad that we end up being separated.
>
> I was a teacher and had children - why can't someone teach me what I'm doing wrong? Dad scolded me all my life if I ever did anything wrong and now I feel as if I've done something wrong.
>
> I guess it's just as well for me to have it as someone else. I know it's sad.

June 17, 1989

We have been away for the Baptist Convention in Ottawa and then I was away for three days at the Cabinet Retreat – the administrative board of the Bible College and Seminary. Mom only asked once where we were – she asked Darrell where his parents were and when I came home she had no sense that I'd been away for longer than my usual day at work, although she asked me if I saw anything in the "east" that I liked better than what we had in the west. It apparently registered that I went to Ottawa, and of course, most of the time she thinks we're in the west. It has relieved my mind considerably to know that she won't fret when I'm away and so I can actually look forward to our trip to England. She was terribly agitated when we went to Oregon, and the agitation was even more intense when we came home and it lasted for a good month or more. She seems to be less concerned with where Fred is now, although it still surfaces from time to time.

> Lesson Learned: Time eventually becomes meaningless.

7. Missed Clues

Summer 1989

We had some moments of panic – and yet in the midst of it something to laugh about. The phone rang in the middle of the night and it was Ruth in BC saying, "Lynn, don't panic! But the police have Mom!!" I bounded out of bed to Mom's room and there was her bed all neatly made up. At midnight, she had dressed, and headed out to go home which she always believed was just around the corner. However, it wasn't, and so she rang a doorbell. The man who answered realized she was confused and called the police who took her to the various seniors' residences to see if she had wandered from there, then took her to the police station and called all the Adcocks in the phone book. No one was missing a grandmother. Finally, she said she was going to visit her son in BC and so they called the only Adcock in BC and reached Ruth who gave them our address. When the police brought her back home, Mom thought she was just coming to visit, had been at the train station and, pointing to the police officer, asked me to pay this nice taxi driver for bringing her home. Then she looked around for her suitcase. I thought quickly and said, "Oh, that was sent on ahead and it's already in your room." She happily headed off upstairs to bed. The police came back the next day to see that she was okay. These recurring notes were the warnings I didn't recognize!!!

Dear Lynn and family -   I am planning on taking a few clothes and going to visit John and Ruth. I need family - why should I be alone? Where is Fred?

Do tell me what and why -I love my family and need their advice and love, Mom

---

to Dad,

Hi - I'm really homesick so want to go home as soon as possible -   Please tell me when it is best to leave to get home so that I'm not doing anything wrong - Thanks M.F.A.

It is not quite "8" but I am going to bed - Please wake me to get up in the morning -- I would like to go North in the morning to see my family - M.F.A.

Fred, will you please meet me at the bus tonight?

I need to go home and visit family - I need to talk to you so please talk and help me over this mountain – it is too big for me to go alone – love Mom (I do need love) and need your advice and help. I need you now – Mom A Frances

Why am I lonely and worried sick?

Perhaps someone is trying to be funny" but it is a queer way of having fun.

Please help me to get away tomorrow — packing etc; I'll need help — thank you
Gram + Mom A.

Lesson Learned: Put an alarm on your door and get an identification bracelet before you need it.

August 18, 1989

Dear Fred,

I don't understand why but I haven't had a word (a letter) or anything from you Why? You have written to the others so they say but I have had no word or letter and wonder what I have done to not deserve even a word. Why why why – has my pension been cut from you?

This is a lonely place and not being used to being alone, it is really lonely.

I would like to find something to do to keep busy and not feel alone. In fact I will "have" to find something – I have kept busy all my life, so it is hard to do "nothing"

Why do you not write? I do not understand your attitude – it seems inhuman and "a push" out into the world.

If you want nothing to do with me, I can do nothing about it – (I did the best I could by my teacher's salary) but that is gone – You cannot get any more now from the pension as I understand –

I am happy with my pension and willing to share – just be glad we have a little pension – we won't starve. M.F.A

Sept 6, 1989 To John and Ruth Adcock and Family -- Please find me - I need family now. Dear Family, I need you now. I need someone to tell me how I got here and where should I go to see all my family - it is rather scary to be so alone and not know where to find anyone. Please help. I can do a lot of things yet but need someone to talk and tell me what to do. Love Mom A.

This is Lynn's home and I live here with them - I don't have to leave and I feel safe and not alone.

Please tell <u>John and Ruth</u> to come to visit - I need my <u>whole family.</u> Please come - where did Fred go? I want to visit with him - I need to visit with him now. Please - and why not -- I love you all. Why should I not love <u>all</u> my family. Return this ---- to John and Ruth and family today - <u>Why</u> do they not come to visit anymore.

Please find Fred and tell him where I am - and **tell me**

LYNN I NEED YOU NOW - something is really wrong

September 19, 1989

I really should be keeping a diary in order to be able to help others through this maze of conflicting emotions.

Sept 22/89
Will you Please waken us when you come alive in the morning - I need to <u>get going</u> - somehow somewhere----M.F.A.

DARRELL please don't let your parents get away tomorrow before we find out whose (wedding day) or what or what or when -

We need to know where and what - (Re pictures on the wall etc etc -) We all need to think <u>THINK</u>

January 7, 1990

I have not been able to write - I have scarcely been able to live.

Mom and I both got the flu at the beginning of December. I'm not fully over it – have a cough still – but although Mom has no signs of cough or cold, she has never come back to the level she was before she got sick. I'm not sure she ever will. She has been with us for over a year now, and we are able to see significant deterioration. She is quite unable to follow any instructions – she can't figure out how to set the table any more, where to find the milk, how to get upstairs, where she should sleep. She asks constantly when she should be going home and how she's going to get there. Last night, after I told her she was to sleep in her own room upstairs, she wandered around for a while quite lost and then came back to ask if she should go up the stairs in the middle of the house, or if she should use the outside stairs!!! I have no idea if she ever lived in a house with outside stairs! It is so very sad.

The notes are increasing in urgency.

> My shopping bag and all its contents were taken from outside my door last evening - some study books and bits of this and that in a sort of "shopping bag" M.F.A. Next room to office - There were study books etc.

> Lynn - I need to talk to you or some understanding person - NOW
> I need to know about so many things and I will need help, re banking etc -
> - I need to know so much
> --tomorrow will do
> (I think)
> Something has gone wrong

> I need to go home - NOW
> In fact I <u>should</u> go now.

> To Lynn -
> Please tell me why I am here and have several pictures here - - I need to know many things about me and why etc etc. etc. -

> I need these books <u>now</u>
> I need to know when and where the family are <u>now</u>
> We need to get together, <u>now</u>

> I need to know about the bank.

> Dear Lynn and family
> Why am I still here - Why shouldn't I go home? Why Why-Love Frances
> (Please talk to me)

8. Added Assistance

January 19, 1990

I went out to Victoria over the New Year for Karen's wedding. It was a good break for me – 5 days – and I realize that I need those kinds of short breaks now and again as long as I have Mom here. I had reached the point of having nothing to give – and just needed some space and some fun. I am trying to get a girl or woman in on a fulltime basis – to live in – in addition to Marcia who comes in the daytime. In exchange for room and board, she could give me some freedom to get out. A student would be ideal because her hours would be flexible.

February 4, 1990

Dad is doing really well. He plans to come down here for their 60th wedding anniversary in July – but I am not planning a big event because he really isn't sure he WILL come. George Sager has a sister near here who also has Alzheimer Disease and is planning to come so they may travel together which would be really good for them both. We'll have to wait and see.

(*Postscript 2014* Dad didn't come then but did come for Mom's 90th birthday in March 1991.)

February 22, 1990

Last night Mom asked me where Lynn was. I didn't answer immediately, waiting to see if she was going to recognize me, or realize that she meant someone else. She asked me then why I was looking at her so strangely. I said, "Well, I'm Lynn!" It took a moment to register and then she laughed and said, "Oh, of course, I know you're Lynn, but I meant the other Lynn, MY Lynn!" I suppose she was looking for an 11 year old!! Poor soul. Julie and Dave were here on Saturday and Mom asked Julie if she'd left her mother home alone. We tried to get her to understand that

I was her mother but she just couldn't comprehend that at all – so the connections are getting more and more fragile.

We have a girl, Linda – a student from the seminary – living with us now and it's helping to give us some more freedom to get out, and it will help me even more when I'm able to drive again. Since I broke my wrist, Linda has been my chauffeur which has been marvelous but I can't wait to be independent again!!

May 19, 1990

Mom was up in the night opening doors and turning on lights in our room and Linda's room. When I said, "Mom, it's the middle of the night and people are sleeping!!" she replied, "What difference does that make when I don't know where anybody is!"

June 20 1990

Mom found me in my study at 11:10 this morning.

"Oh you're here. I was wanting to go to the kitchen. How do I find it?"

"You just go down those steps."

"Down those steps and turn at the bottom?"

"Yes, are you wanting some breakfast?"

"Oh, I wasn't thinking about breakfast. I just wanted to find them and say thank you."

"Thank you for what?

"They sent me a note – Gayle and Gerry – when their colts died (near tears) *– they were so*

> June 25, 1990
> Please, don't go away and leave me alone -- anywhere. <u>Mom A</u>
> <u>Don't forget.</u> I'm upstairs and alone--- M.F.A. <u>I need to go home.</u>

thoughtful. I don't know how they got the news - I don't know how anybody knows anything.....you asked about breakfast. Do they serve breakfast here?"

July 1, 1990

I am going to Denver for a conference next week. Roger is flying out at the end of the conference and we'll take a car and go into the mountains for a few days. We need a break with no responsibilities for a while.

Mom enjoys Alicia a lot although she isn't always sure who she belongs to. She knows she fits into the family somewhere but isn't sure where.

Mom's doctor told me there is a drug – I didn't write down the name so I have to wait until I see him again to get it – that is now available through Ottawa for Alzheimer's patients. It is a calcium channel blocker which prevents calcium (and aluminum, apparently) from entering the cells. Most victims seem to have excess calcium and aluminum stored in their brain cells. There is a natural process by which cells get rid of the calcium and if that is still intact, then the prevention of any further "getting in" should gradually improve their functioning. If it is the "getting rid of it" process that is not functioning, then preventing more from entering will not improve the condition but should at least prevent it from getting worse. The drug has been approved in the states but it is only available in Canada for research purposes. The side effects are not well known yet, but I'd like to put Mom on it anyway because she is continuing to deteriorate and if there is anything that would help, it would be worth the risk. The doctor is going to try to get authority from Ottawa and will call me when he has some word – he thought maybe 10 days.

(*Postscript 2014* He never did get approval – at least in time for Mom.)

I had an assessment for Mom for respite care and long term care on Tuesday. I have booked two weeks in January for her to go into the Cummer Lodge where she goes to the day care once a week. Roger and I will probably go south then for a holiday. Also, it will put her on the waiting list for the residence. She has gone down hill in the last few months quite a bit and the drug may not help. In many ways she's still doing really well. She is still up and active almost all day and sleeps well at night. She can socialize well and enjoys getting out. I took her to get flowers for the garden and you'd never know she's 89. She isn't fretting as much about going home as she used to although she still asks almost every day how she can get home, and where Fred is. Most of the time, I'm her sister and we grew up in the same home on the farm!! Sometimes she asks about visiting her parents, often she wants to go to John and Ruth's – or she wants to phone them to come for her. Sometimes she looks at the house and tells me it's just like where we used to live – it even has a pond in the back like at home (that's our backyard pool!!) sometimes it's "just like Lynn's only there aren't as many trees as at Lynn's!!" She just can't keep it sorted out, but she seems more content most of the time than she was for quite a while. The agitation and intensity has diminished considerably, and her weepy periods are farther apart - so we're doing okay most of the time.

> July 1990
>
> I am going home in the morning. The cows and calves and chickens are more company and have more friends that one does here. Bye now - will see you when I get up in the morning - bye now
>
> I will not be staying here - it is so lonely and dreary. I can come and get my clothes someday soon - there are places and other ways of getting educated. I will try them. It is more lonely here than on the farm. The animals there will talk to anyone. I will come and talk to you some day again. It is bedtime now - As ever Frances Adcock

July 25, 1990

Julie and Dave were here for Sunday with all the family, and then stayed for another day. Julie and I went shopping. On Tuesday morning Julie's birthday cake was sitting on the table and Mom asked about it.

> *"That's the rest of Julie's Birthday cake."*
> *"Was she here?"*
> *"Yes, we were all together for a big party on Sunday?"*
> *"Was I here, too?"*
> *"Yes, you were here."*
> *"Were Julie's parents here?"*
> *"I'm Julie's Mom."*

Sept 16, 1990

Why am I alone? I have many friends and relatives, so why am I here alone? I need my family -
Please tell me what has happened to my family - I need my friends and family <u>now</u>. I must find them as soon as possible - M F. (Hoover) (gone to bed) alone and disgusted

---

October 1, 1990

At four o'clock this morning Mom came to our room. She sometimes comes to check if anyone is there, thinking she's all alone, but this time she was trying to find her own room. She had gotten up to the bathroom and couldn't find her room. The light was off in her room so I don't know if she had turned off the light when she left the room or if she had decided it wasn't hers and then turned it off. I told her I'd take her back and showed her to her room, then headed back to bed. A few minutes later I saw the light again, got up and found her out in the hall. I asked her, "What's the matter?" and she said she had to find out where she was, that that wasn't her room. She turned the light on in my office and said, "Oh that's the office, but where's my room?" I ushered her into her room, assured her it was her room and she said, "Are you sure?" Then she saw the picture on the wall of her and Dad and said, "Oh yes, there's that picture, and then spying her suitcase which she had been packing, said, "And there's my suitcase. What's it doing there? I guess I must have been packing." Thinking quickly, I said, "No, I think you just didn't finish getting it unpacked." I wasn't about to reinforce the idea that she was going somewhere. I managed to get her to climb into bed and then I turned out the light. I went back to bed but didn't get back to sleep again. I think I kept expecting her to get up again.

I have noticed quite a deterioration recently, although it was amazing to see her be the life of the party when Linda had some friends over. No one would ever have known there was anything wrong with her except that I knew that some of the information she gave was mixed up. But it was surprising to have her not recognize her room. She often doesn't know that she has a room upstairs but when she comes up, has up 'til now had no difficulty recognizing it as hers.

> Lesson Learned: One of the realities of the loss of memory is losing the ability to visualize what is out of sight, very much like a 2 year old who hasn't yet learned that what is out of sight still exists. That explains her inability to know what is downstairs – and where we are when we're in another room – and where her own room is. And as soon as others are out of sight she feels alone. While it made me sad, I realized I couldn't do anything to change that.

Tonight she wanted to phone Fred again. She said she needed a man to look after her – that she guessed she had never told him that – that she probably had treated him in an offhand way so he thought she didn't need him. And that he needed her, too. A husband and wife should be together.

Then later she asked me if I didn't have room for her to sleep here tonight.

> *"You have your own room here. Why would you think there wasn't any room?"*
> *"Well, you never said anything about inviting me so I thought you mustn't have room for me."*
> *"Mom, I didn't say anything because it's your own room and you can go there anytime you want."*
> *"Well, I didn't say anything because I don't want to be hoggish about my room."*

She then said, "I thought we would have time for a short visit, but I guess we don't so I'll just go on upstairs." I had been counseling someone and she was left to sit with Roger watching the ball game. I guess she thought she had come to visit me and I didn't have time for her.

> Lesson Learned: I learned that the loss of memory includes the loss of a sense of time. So leaving Mom alone for 5 minutes was not that different in her mind than when we were away for 5 days.

January 13, 1991

This is Sunday Morning – Mom wouldn't/couldn't get going for church this morning so I am home. I am at that waiting stage – waiting for a phone call from Julie to say that her baby is on the way. I'm hoping that the call won't come until after Wednesday, though, because Mom is going into the nursing home for three weeks to give me some flexibility to be there for Julie. I am really looking forward to this time partly because I am in need of a break and partly because it's a once in a lifetime experience for mother and daughter to be together for her first baby. I just hope it all works out with my school schedule as well. There are so many things that I can't control – so it all has to be left in God's hands, and I have to accept what comes.

Our Christmas was fairly quiet in the sense that I didn't do any entertaining apart from immediate family. I began to wonder how I managed to do all the entertaining I used to do and realized that when the children were all at home, we were one unit and so it was easy to reach out to two or three other units and interact with them. The children were just a part of the core. Now that they are separate units, they become the two or three other units that I reach out to – and try to co-ordinate with – and it becomes more complicated. All my energy, which isn't what it used to be, is used up with my own children. I am beginning to see how families can get inward looking – or perhaps it's better to say, how they can fail to be outward looking. I'm not laying any guilt on myself for this – it's just helpful to understand what's happening. I don't expect that I will have the kind of energy it takes to do my old kind of entertaining as long as I have Mom living here. This is the "stage of life" I am at right now and that's okay.

Mom continues to get more and more confused. She had a bout of shingles this fall and then fell and cracked her rib – so it has not been a good few months. Every day by late afternoon as she sees it getting dark she is wanting to go home before it gets dark. Then when it is dark, she is so worried about how she will get home, and worried that "they" will be worried about her not being home before dark. I explain to her that she is home, that this is where she lives, that she doesn't need to go anywhere, that we are family. And she is so relieved. She wants to know where she can sleep and how to find her room and says that it is so good to know that she doesn't have to leave. Then she will look at the window and say, "It's really black out there," and start the whole thing again. She can sometimes be distracted but not usually for very long.

One morning recently after being up in the night with her, trying to get her settled down and listening to her sob in her terrible loneliness and confusion, she said, "Lynn doesn't have time to talk to me. She's just so busy all the time." I said, "I'm Lynn and I'm here to talk to you." She looked at me, trying to sort out what I said and then laughed and repeated her familiar phrase, "Oh, of course, I know you're Lynn, but I mean MY Lynn." And last night when she came to the table to sit at the same place she's occupied for two years, she talked about this new place and how nice it was of me to give her something to eat – and then went into the whole business again about how was she going to get home. Last Sunday at lunch, she kept talking about how nice it was of the lady who owns this place to leave things out for us just to help ourselves like this and kept wondering how I had managed to make arrangements with her. And so it goes!

March 1991

Mom's 90th Birthday was a wonderful celebration. Gayle, John and Ruth, her brother Roy and wife Win, and Dad all came and we took lots of pictures which she has enjoyed. She was content and basked in all the attention. Something about having Fred beside her was familiar but I'm pretty sure she thought he was her Dad not her husband. It didn't really matter – Fred was here – and it made her happy. We all had a chuckle when Dad walked through the door and was greeted with Mom's, "Well, it's about time you came home!!"

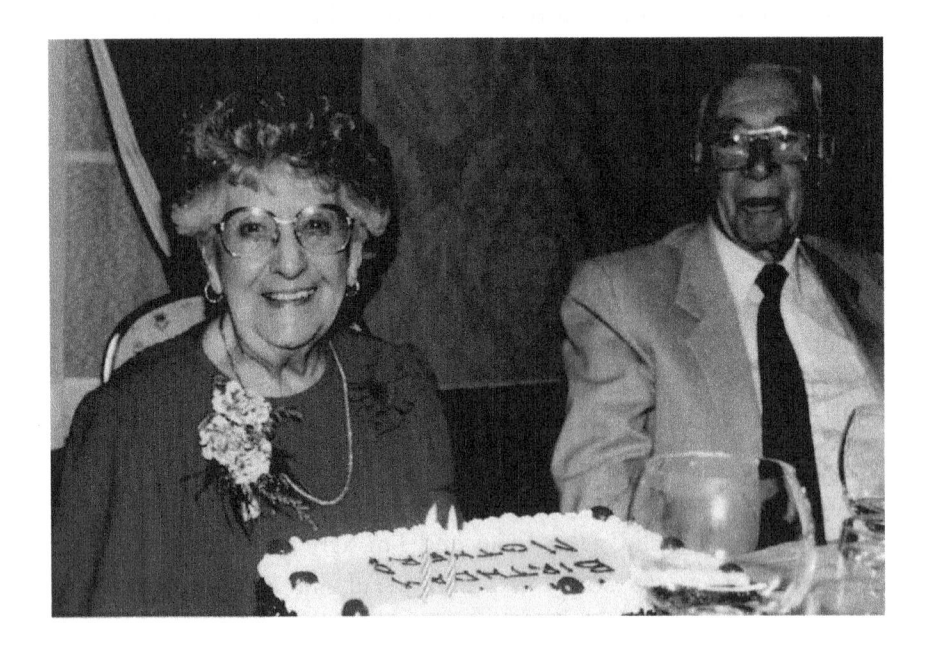

B. The Nursing Home

1. Another Trauma

Separating Mom from Dad by bringing her to Toronto was a difficult decision – but we knew it was necessary. A much harder decision was moving her to a nursing home – perhaps because I couldn't be sure it was necessary.

I knew I could not continue indefinitely and eventually it would be necessary to move Mom into a home – but when? It took a long time for me to make that decision and an even longer time for the pain of that decision to subside. How desperately I needed the counsel of someone who had walked that road before me who might have helped me sort out what's true and what's false so that I could stand up against the inner accusations. At the core of my being I knew that I could not continue much longer – but Mom was getting old and I kept thinking I can manage another 6 months. Had I known she would live another 7 years, perhaps the decision may not have been so difficult for it would have been obvious to me that I couldn't continue for that long. I say, "Perhaps," because how can I know? I only know that the decision was agonizing.

May 16, 1991

Dear Dad, Gayle and Gerry, John and Ruth,

I would have phoned you but I have no voice and so it would make explanations very difficult, especially to you, Dad. (Explanation - Dad was hard of hearing so telephone calls were difficult.) *So I decided to write one letter and copy it to all of you. The news is that Mom is now in a nursing home. What happened was that I called to arrange some respite care for myself for over the summer or in September when I have such a busy schedule and was told that the respite care subsidy had been taken away by the government in February. I had just made it for January! That really threw me as it would cost $55.00 a day to have her stay there and I would need to keep Marcia on at $64.00 a day – an expensive holiday just to stay home!!*

Then when I asked some more questions, I discovered that they are ready to start renovations fairly quickly and they will take about a year to complete. The message I got was that if I didn't place her pretty quickly, I may not get her in for a year because they will need to clear out a whole wing at a time to do the renovations, so they will be reducing their numbers starting any time now.

I had looked at a number of places again after you were all here for her Birthday, and it just confirmed for me that Cummer Lodge was the only choice, albeit not what I would have liked for her. She is not able to go into the many "Homes for the Aged" which are generally much nicer because she has to be able to live independently when she goes in. Once she was in, they would keep her even if she became bed-ridden, but no one would take her as she is. The other extreme is the nursing home and they, too, are much nicer, but there isn't the same level of activity available as the funding is much less so the staff ratio isn't as high. The one place that I would have liked her to go (Where I took you, Ruth) was lovely but they only took people from the hospitals. However, what that place gave me was an idea of what Cummer Lodge will look like when they do the renovations and that helped make me feel a little better.

It was not an easy decision – I think my sore throat is a result of two nights of walking the floor. I knew that I could not manage for another year, and yet I wasn't happy putting her in such an old building. All the newer ones were so far away that visiting would be less likely to happen spontaneously. Cummer Lodge is close to my work so I can pop over at lunch or on the way home from work and see her often. Also, it will be easy for our kids to stop by when they come, or for us to bring her here so she'll get to see the great-grandchildren often.

Julie went with me to see the room and she figured she could have a full time job just wandering around with Lindsay. They were all so happy to see a baby. At the moment Mom is in a room with four – but when the renovations are done they will be all single and double rooms. One lady in with her, Mabel, is just a sweetheart and was so glad to have Mom come so she could have someone to talk to. She has three daughters who are all school teachers and so she and Mom hit it off right away. The other two ladies in the room (one had her 100th Birthday in November) are physically well, too, and are always out in the lounge but they aren't talkative enough for Mabel.

We've taken in some pictures, a new white dresser to replace the hospital style one they use and I am looking for a chair that will match the colours in the room to give her some "esthetics".

She's quite happy not to be in a room alone as she often fretted about that here. But she knows she's in a "place" rather than at home...although she thought she was in some sort of "place" here, too, a lot of the time.

Marcia was not very happy with me. I had told her back in April that I was considering it and that I would pay her until the end of May. She kept saying, "You don't have to take it. You can just tell them you're still managing!" Well, when I told her, we both had a good bawl. She said, "But she's my Mom!"

I can't tell you I am happy about my decision. I wish I had never had to make it, and it's hard every time I go to see her, because she hates to see me leave. But I <u>can</u> say that I'm glad I brought her here to Toronto, because she's had two really good years with us. I said that when the time came for me to put Mom into a home, it would be for <u>me</u> and that I wouldn't try to convince myself that it was for her. That is what it has come to. I am really tired. It was fine when Marcia was with her in the daytime, but she went home to her own space and I took over. Marcia was right – I could have managed a while longer, but not without respite and not indefinitely. And so the decision I had to make was, would it be now, or could I risk it being another year? I chose now - rather than letting myself get totally worn out.

It would be best to send any mail for her to me and I'll take it over because she puts things away and then forgets she got them. She has a bulletin board so I can pin up cards or pictures. As soon as I get everything fixed up for her, I'll take a picture so you have a sense of where she is.

It was hard – and still is. When I took her back tonight after being out in Hamilton, she couldn't understand why she was there and why I was leaving and why I was leaving her and why Fred wasn't there etc. etc.

July 1991

When I visit Mom, I never know who I am in her eyes until I am leaving. I walk away slowly so that I can listen. With her social graces still intact, she will turn to the woman sitting next to her and say, "That woman is….." And then I know if I have been her sister, mother, friend or someone she taught with years ago. I don't recall ever being called her daughter. Occasionally she would ask if I had see Lynn recently. Clearly she was looking for the child she remembered.

57

One day, her words took me totally by surprise as she explained to her neighbor, "That woman is married to my son-in-law!!"

It reminded me of the message her doctor gave me about patients with dementia. He said, "There's no way of knowing when something will connect and when it won't." He likened it to having a tray full of light bulbs all partially screwed in to their sockets. Each time you shake the tray, different lights would come on randomly and there's no way of predicting which connections will be made at any given time. We saw evidence of that time and time again.

When her sister Grace died, I wasn't sure if I should tell her or if it would even register. I chose to tell her and there was no indication that the message registered at the time. However, many months later, she told me that Grace had died and she couldn't figure out why no one in the family had told her.

August 18, 1991

Mom seems to be adjusting to the home – she used to be really emotional when I arrived and worse when I left – now she is just pleasantly surprised to see me and more accepting of my departure. It is still hard when I bring her home and then take her back. That's the time she is most upset. She introduces me as her little sister to all the rest of the ladies! And she's very confused about where she is, but then she was confused when she was here, too.

> Lesson Learned: Dementia is different from normal forgetfulness – something I need to remind myself of every time I forget something.

2. The Difficult Decisions Continue

February 19, 1992

Dear Brenda,

I want to apologize for taking so long to respond to the good news that you are being married next summer – and to let you know officially that we will definitely be there. I had a hard time when your Mom called to tell me because I had promised that I'd bring Grandma out for your wedding and it broke my heart to think that I couldn't keep that promise. So, as you can guess, I cried.

The truth is that she would be so confused that she would not be able to enter in to the celebration. When she can visit for short periods of time, she is just fine, but she needs to know where she is and how she got there whenever she is in unfamiliar surroundings. We bring her home for all the celebrations that we have – and we celebrate everything! – but it's really difficult for her to keep us all straight and to know why she's here and Fred isn't!!

Your Mom said that you'd had your cry too, but that she convinced you that it would be better to remember her as she was and that your Mom wants to remember her as she was on her Birthday as well...that you would find it difficult to see her confused.

It was fun to look at all the pictures your Mom sent to Grandma. And having everything labeled for Grandma is just wonderful. It was the first time I'd seen a picture of Gord so now we know who you're marrying!! Pretty neat looking guy, I'd say!! Is he as nice as he looks? Hope so.

We certainly wish you all the best and we're looking forward to being there for your special day. We're not sure yet when we are coming out, nor what route we'll take when we get there, but we want to see everyone so that means Edmonton, Calgary, the Okanagan, Merritt, Kamloops and the Cariboo. It's too bad we can't stay long enough to be there for Brad's wedding, too, but we'll at least get to meet Cindy.

Happy planning – see you in August!

Love Auntie Lynn and Uncle Roger

September 5, 1992

Mom is in great shape and she is quite content. She's still delighted to see me, but since I've been away, she just doesn't seem to have the same kind of recognition as before. I thought at first I might be imagining it but then I spoke to a lady at church on Sunday who takes her out quite often and she said the same thing as I've been feeling since I got back. She had been away for a few weeks as well so it may be that the familiarity will come back with regular visits. Of course, it may be that she's just lost that much more of her memory and I don't notice the change as much when I see her often. She still covers her confusion really well!! I had her to the eye clinic last week and she has cataract surgery scheduled for Oct 21st. They'll take off the one on her left eye which is totally solid now, because the right one is growing fairly quickly and it may need to be done within the next year as well. It will depend on how good her vision is after this one is done.

3. Surgery and Unexpected Consequences

October 25, 1992

On Wednesday Mom had her cataract surgery. I picked her up at 6 am to have her there for 6:30. Surgery was at 8 and it went well. I sent her back in the Cummer Lodge bus because I was really afraid of my driving being too jerky just after surgery. I was able to use my right foot for the gas but still was braking with my left foot. (I had sprained my right ankle.) When she arrived she had pulled the patch off her eye. I had known that she wouldn't remember what the patch was for and would need to be constantly told that she had had surgery, but it never occurred to me that she would actually pull it off. It was something I just hadn't anticipated and I didn't know what to do. I just felt sick every time I thought about her rubbing her eye. So I finally decided the only solution was to arrange an around the clock watch with a combination of paid and volunteer help. One of the women in the church took on the responsibility of phoning a number of people and the schedule was all filled in except for this Friday morning and I was free to sit with her. I worked at her table during the times when she slept.

I'm hoping that by Wednesday night she'll be past the danger stage. I have a conference that I am the MC for that starts on Thursday and goes through to Saturday noon so I have a lot to do this week in preparation. Had I known that this was going to happen, I would have postponed the surgery until next week. Hindsight is wonderful isn't it!!

Written to those who sat with Mom

Dear ....

I am writing to say a very special thank you for your willingness to be a part of the team who saw Mom through her "eye patch" week. I had anticipated the fact that she would need to be reminded constantly that she had a patch on her eye because she had just had a cataract removed, but it simply did not occur to me that she would take the patch off – although in retrospect, I realize that's perfectly reasonable!! Had I thought, I would not have chosen the week before a big conference to have her surgery!!

The doctor is pleased and once she has her new glasses, she will be in good shape – and I owe you a great debt of gratitude.

Several things have happened as a result of having so many people go in. One is that you were all a witness to the nurses of the kind of care a Christian community provides. Another is that your perspective on Mom has helped me see her in a new light. I have seen her through the eyes of history and that has meant missing the person she was – the woman who was once so capable and competent and independent and my friend as well as my mother – and I have grieved. But many of you who sat with her told me of sensing her peace and of finding yourselves quieter and calmer for having been with her and I have come to realize that instead of being the "nothing" I see because of what she has lost, she is still somebody and her presence is still able to have an impact for good. She can still be a blessing. And that realization is a wonderful gift to me.

So not only have you helped keep her eyesight, you have given me a new vision of my mother – and I am so grateful to you.

November 3, 1992

Dear Dad,

I have an envelope around here somewhere that has been here a long time so I decided I should get some things into it and send it away. A letter is one of the "things"!!

I've just written a whole pile of thank you notes to those who sat with Mom and then thought that you might like to see the list that was in place for the week. Some of them are ones I needed to hire – particularly through the night, and for the first few days to give me a chance to get things in place. The rest are either students from the seminary or women from the church. It's interesting how many of them came back to me with comments of appreciation. One student had been doing her field placement there and had not known that Mom was there. She had not been happy going because she hadn't been able to connect with anyone and had found it depressing but just spending time with Mom transformed her whole outlook on visiting the women there. Now she's excited about going and keeps thanking me for asking her.

One of the women from the church said she found herself slowing down and talking softer and ended up feeling calmer and gentler and again thanked me. Another felt a real sense of peace being with her and commented on how different she is from so many in there who are agitated and angry. She, too, came away feeling better for having been there.

It was good for me to get the perspective of others because I am more inclined to see what's missing – her vitality and initiative and ability to enter into other people's worlds. They see her graciousness and gentleness in what I see as passivity. The realization that others can still receive from her – that they can experience her as a blessing in the midst of what I see as her "nothingness" has been a wonderful gift to me. I still grieve whenever I see her, but I am better able to see her value – to accept who she is right now – and not think that because so much is gone, that she's totally gone. She would be thrilled, I know, if she could understand that she is still able to be an avenue of blessing.

November 8, 1992

Mom now sees clearly from the operated eye – last time things were still a little blurry and when I spoke to the doctor he said her eye was still swollen somewhat so I was really glad when she said she could see clearly from that eye. The other one is cloudy because the cataract is growing quickly in it but at this point, I'm just glad to have her have one good eye. She goes to get tested for glasses on Tuesday so we'll see then what the doctor says. He has been very good about going to the home to see her and is always quite willing to talk to me when I call so I am grateful. Most ophthalmologists would be too busy to be bothered.

January 19, 1993

Mom is pretty much the same. Her cataract operation has been successful and so her eyesight is so very much improved. It seemed to make her brighter and more alert – like maybe some of the confusion of her world was that everything was seen through a cataract fog!

January 28, 1993

Mom is fine, although I haven't seen her for a week because the lodge is under quarantine because of a flu outbreak. This is the second time since she's been there that they've quarantined the place. It seems to just spread right through in spite of the fact that they all get flu shots every fall.

June 14, 1993

Mom is well - doesn't seem to change much these days – at least not in any dramatic way. Over the months as I look back I can see that the changes have been there but they are very gradual. Usually I am her sister, but this week I was her niece. At least I am still family and that means a lot to her.

4. Where's Fred?

July 16, 1995

I have just come back from the family picnic at Cummer lodge. It's interesting how, as soon as we get into a group of people, Mom looks around wondering, "Where's Fred?"

October 14, 1995

Mom fell and badly gashed her arm about two weeks ago now but it's healing up quite nicely. This is about the third time she has fallen in the last year and the amazing thing is that she hasn't broken any bones. Her legs aren't as strong as they were because she isn't getting the exercise she needs and when she gets up from a chair she uses her arms to pull herself up rather than her legs – so I'm not sure what happens when she falls and of course she doesn't remember falling so you can't find out from her. My concern is that she'll break a hip and be bedridden. She's still fairly active and it would be hard for her to lose her ability to be independently mobile. She's quite something, though, in that she still has her delightful sense of humour.

I took in a bunch of deep red maple leaves yesterday. She has all her meals with the same group of women who are all quite sociable and so they all enjoy anything I take in. I often time my visits so that I can get her settled at the lunch or dinner table before I leave. Then she's not so concerned about my leaving.

January 1996

Mom enjoyed her Christmas with us. She remains about the same.

When Mom lived with us, she spent her whole time with us attempting to "go home" if only I'd help her get there and sometimes she would set out on her own. The longer she stayed and the more advanced her dementia became, the younger she became in her mind, and therefore the mental picture of "home" eventually became the farm in Saskatchewan where she grew up. Once she was in the nursing home, that drive to "go home" seemed to vanish.

I learned today that it is perhaps because the memory became the reality. The nursing home has become the farm home.

She was so excited and wanted to show me around the place they had just bought. All the bedrooms meant that all the family could come at once and there would be room for everyone. She kept talking about what a good deal they had made. We looked out the window at the bush next to the lodge and she commented that there was still a lot of work to be done – all the bush needed to be cleared, but they had good horses and lots of help and so they would be able to do it. It was indeed a good deal. I couldn't help but think how deeply rooted our basic values really are. They seem to survive even the onslaught of something like Alzheimer's and provide meaning to life even when it appears meaningless to others. I am often so sad that she can't enjoy the connections that we are making with family when that is so important to her. And yet it seems as if her spirit and what's left of her mind create illusions that allow her to rejoice in what she holds dear anyway. And so in the midst of my sadness, I enter into her world and rejoice with her. And I'm so glad God has given me the ability to do that. Just wish I had learned that sooner.

I am planning to have an open house for Mom on March 31st. Her Birthday happens to land on a Sunday which makes it perfect. There are a number of women in the church who have been incredibly kind to Mom over the years. It's hard to believe she has been here over seven years now. Anyway, I'd like to have them in to give Mom the occasion to thank them as well as to honour Mom on her Birthday.

Mom still looks for "Fred" whenever she's here. At Christmas, she kept fretting over the fact that Dad was missing out on all the wonderful things. And when she decided it was time to go home, she fully expected him to come for her and kept asking when she should be calling him.

August 1996

Mom said, "Do I have a mama? I need a mama. I need to know what to do and she'll tell me."

Summer 1997

What I had feared might happen *has* happened. Mom fell and broke her hip. When the nurses in the hospital would tell Mom not to try to get out of bed without help, I began to realize how very little they understood about dementia. Did they really think she would remember why she was there, let alone that she shouldn't try to get up? We just made sure she wasn't alone.

She is now in a wheel chair and can't understand the need to experience the pain of standing up to do the therapy required to get her mobile.

February 1, 1998

When Mom broke her second hip – a fracture not a dislocation – I decided that she shouldn't have surgery since it was not going to help her be mobile again anyway as she was already confined to a wheelchair and it seemed cruel to put her through the agony and fear of another hospital stay and the pain of the surgery. In retrospect, it was a good decision. She would not likely have survived the surgery as without adequate exercise, her heart was beginning to fail.

She had to stay in bed until her hip healed and that confused her because she associated being in bed with being sick – or, as I discovered one day - with having a baby. She kept asking where they had taken her baby – saying over and over again, "I love her, I love her."

5. The Final Journey Home

March 1, 1998

I happened to be visiting Mom when the nurses came to change her. Until then I had been praying in my head for God to take her home but hearing her cry of pain as the staff moved her in bed changed that. That day I cried from the depths of my being for God to take her home. Death would be so merciful – such a blessing – for her. A few days later her heart gave out and she died peacefully on the 21st of February.

Each of the three grandchildren spoke at her funeral and so did I. I didn't realize until it was all over that I had done what I needed to do in my eulogy and that was to let people know that the woman they knew in the last 9 years was not the real Frances. I wanted them to know a little of the person I knew. I was quite surprised that I was able to speak and not break – especially after both Julie and Darrell broke down. We had all written out what we wanted to say. Malcolm was first and he got through his okay. Julie had Dave stand beside her so that if she couldn't finish it, he would take over. She couldn't and he did. Then Darrell followed and he had a really hard time getting through his. At one point, he kind of looked around helplessly and then pulled himself together and finished. He told us later that he said to himself, "I wrote this and I'm going to say it!" Then I had to follow him and was quite amazed that I didn't choke up at all. What we all ended up saying – in different ways – was that Mom, or Grandma, had been trying to get "home" for a long time and now she was home – with her mind back, not confused, not wondering where she is, not feeling abandoned – and we rejoiced with her. Darrell's observation was quite interesting in that he said that most people lost their grandparents when they died, but in a strange way, with her death, he now has his real grandma back. He can now remember her as she was when he was growing up and not how she was in the past few years.

I was not prepared for the huge hole that she left in my life. I thought that having dealt with losing her piece by piece, the final goodbye would be relatively easy – just a relief for her and for me. So I wasn't prepared for the intensity of the loss that I felt. But I came to realize that while I had been losing her gradually as my mother and my friend and the competent "with-it" person she had been, my caring for her had created a different relationship but still a very important one. So the hole had not shrunk in size, it had merely changed shape. And I guess I have experienced at an emotional level what I have known in my head – that losing your mother – the one who gave you life – is never easy even when you have nothing but gratitude that she has come to the end of her suffering and is finally "at home."

We're doing well. It will take a long time to erase the last 9 years. For instance, for the last 6 years, every time I went to and from work, as I went by her corner, I would check my watch to see if there was time to slip in for a quick hello. Every time I went past the flowers in the mall, or grocery store, I would stop and think through the rest of my day to decide if I could take her some. So now, as I pass that corner, I am conscious that she isn't there anymore and as I see the flowers, I'm reminded that I can't take them to her anymore. – sometimes it's just an awareness I have – sometimes it's a sadness I feel –sometimes it's a relief – but always I'm happy that she is no longer the way she was in the last couple of months. Gradually the recent memories are fading and the memories of her long and vibrant life are taking their place. For that I am grateful.

C. Eulogy for Mom

Mom, I know you're not in that box but I'm going to talk to you as if you were there.

Many years ago, now, I was able to convince you that it wasn't any more humble to wear the dark and dull colours that characterized the prairie homesteaders than to wear the bright and vivid colours of God's creation. Your artist's eye took to the colours, even though you often struggled with feeling really bold. I always took great delight in finding you colourful clothes to wear and so today I have had special delight in seeing that your last appearance on earth is in your brightest red dress. If you could see yourself in a mirror, I know I would hear that familiar expression of your not-easily-disguised pleasure, "Not bad for an old lady!"

Mom, I'm so glad that you are at last home. For so many years you were sure that if you just went around the corner you would find your old farm and everything would be just right again because you had found your way home.

You had such determination that it energized you to the point that I had to run to catch up to you when you took off up the street.

But now at last you are home – not to the old farm where things are temporary at best – but to your real home which is forever. There's no more wondering where you are, no more chafing at the imprisonment you felt for so long, no more confusion, and best of all – no more feeling of being abandoned. You are home. We will miss you – but in reality we have been missing you bit by bit for many years now and so it seems like it has taken us a long time to say our goodbyes.

We said goodbye to you in stages.

First we lost the mother and grandmother who was always so interested in all the little things her family was involved in. You became self-focused as you tried to grasp and hang onto the reality that control was slipping away and you didn't know where it was going.

It was painful to watch you grapple with your confusion. It was emotionally draining to try to keep you sorted out. It was sad to watch you lose your dignity, to slop your food. It was painful to think how embarrassed you would be if you had known how you were behaving. It made me angry to see you spoken to crossly because you couldn't cooperate, to be handled less than gently because you couldn't follow directions, to have your fears minimized because you didn't always respond appropriately. I kept wanting to cry out, "You don't know the woman I know." "That's not who she is."

I became acutely aware of the fact that we were losing you.

We lost the mother who exhibited such great courage in the face of difficulty: you became like a frightened child terrified of the unknown, clinging to what was solid and real and secure. You conquered that fear and flew to Toronto on your own to be at Julie's wedding. I told you at that time that you were "one gutsy lady" and you said that was the nicest thing anyone could have said. You saw yourself as a coward all your life because you didn't like being out with the animals on the farm but preferred to be in the kitchen with your mother. You were anything BUT a coward. You were the pioneer in the family – after the pattern of your mother. You headed out for unknown territory time and time again in order to make a better life for yourself and your family.

– Setting out on your own with 3 children to teach in a ten grade one room country school when Dad went into the air force.

– Taking your two young girls on the long train trip from Saskatchewan to British Columbia to teach in an unknown place in order to move the family to a better climate leaving Dad and John to sell the house and move out later.

We lost the mother who had great determination – you became immobilized in your lostness. I have bags full of letters you wrote – notes to various people – many to yourself as you tried to make sense of your confusing world.

We lost the mother whose sense of humour sometimes delightfully shocked us as kids with its earthiness and who could see the funny side of everything. Although one of the recreational assistants at Cummer Lodge commented to me that even when you seemed the most confused, you would occasionally come out with a funny line that made him laugh and we caught glimpses of your humour right up to the end. Our last laugh was over your explanation of your one skinny leg and one swollen one after your broken hip. "The skinny one belongs to me and the fat one belongs to someone else."

We lost the mother who always gave of herself.

We lost the poet. We lost the artist.

We lost the Mother we knew. You became a child looking for your Mama. In your final confusion it was as if you knew only one thing that would make things right – you needed your Mama. And now you are together once again. Her faith instilled in you the truth that this life is not the end but just the beginning.

You loved your great grandchildren's visits – to hold the babies as they came along – and we were sad that you didn't have the full enjoyment of knowing they belonged to you. But we have pictures galore and they will see by the look on your face how much joy they brought to you.

We've said goodbye over the years to pieces of you, Mom. And you didn't know – couldn't comprehend how much you were loved. You just felt abandoned.

We thank you for your courage, your thoughtfulness, your care, your concern, your humour, your wisdom. Thank you for believing in us – each so different and yet so appreciated. Thank you for your simple quiet faith in God that sustained you, and us, through difficult times. You have left us a legacy.

And, Mom, I want to thank you for the gift of your complete acceptance of me. I never had the sense that I had to prove anything to you – it was just fine to be me. You rejoiced with me in my successes, grieved with me in my sorrows, enjoyed my joys. We laughed a lot together, we cried at times together. I sometimes wonder if you laughed with me at the beginning of my life as much as I cried with you at the end of yours.

In my teens, you used to go to bed, but lie awake waiting for me whenever I was out at night to make sure I was home safely before you could go to sleep. I'd come in and sit on your bed and we'd talk - whispering so we wouldn't wake Dad. But we always did.

And now you're once again waiting for me to come home. There will be no more losses, no more goodbyes – only a welcome home. It will be so good to see you again – restored to wholeness and enjoying the fact that you have at last found your way home – home to where you belong, where you know how much you are loved.

You were right, Mom, home <u>was</u> just around the corner and you've made it and everything is now all right.

Good bye, Mom.

We love you. But we need to say goodbye and so we're grateful that God's love is greater than ours. He has not let you go even through your confusion - and He never will.

Hymn - O Love That Will Not Let Me Go.

Section 3 Lessons Learned

There are so many lessons I learned – some very simple practical things to hand on, some more difficult to express, but all a part of the journey.

A. Early Preparation

1. Pay attention to early signs

Without becoming paranoid about forgetfulness, it's wise to pay attention to early signs because it's easier to make decisions about future care <u>with</u> someone than <u>for</u> someone. There are systems that can be put in place more easily when someone is still mentally able to make those decisions. Having someone write out – in their own handwriting so that they recognize it as their own wishes – the kind of care they would like to have could make future decisions easier for everyone. Not every family is able or willing to give the kind of emotional support that I received. How much more difficult it would have been for me if I had to justify every decision I made to the rest of my family. For that I am grateful beyond description.

One of the early signs we had but did not recognize was the day before my niece's wedding in Alberta. Mom was fretting about who was going to drive her to the wedding and whether she would be picked up in time. Julie wrote out all the details for her in a note book which Mom put into her purse. Then she would get up, find her purse, read the note, put it back and sit down again. She must have done that a dozen times. We thought she was just anxious about being dependent on someone else to get her there on time, but looking back we realize that was one of the early signs.

Another sign to pay attention to is the inability to change a mistaken notion. I visited Mom and Dad in Clearbrook and at Mom's suggestion emptied a dresser drawer to use instead of living out of my suitcase. I moved pictures to another drawer and it didn't occur to me to put them back. I just left it empty. Sometime later my Aunt Grace visited. After she left, Mom went looking for something, discovered the empty drawer and was convinced that Grace had stolen her pictures. She wrote nasty letters about Grace to everyone, including the police. Nothing I could say would convince her otherwise. Eventually forgetfulness erases what reason cannot.

Paranoia is another early sign. Mom would hide her rings for fear someone would steal them and then accuse Dad of stealing them. He would spend hours hunting for them – only to have her hide them again.

2. Find a doctor who will listen to your concerns

I think that is easier today than when I visited my mother's doctor with her, but don't let a doctor dismiss your concerns. (April 1989 pp. 34-35)

3. Recognize the uniqueness of dementia

Caring for someone with dementia is very different from caring for someone who is eventually getting better, or someone with physical disabilities, or for a child who is developing. (March 1989 p. 34; October 1990 pp. 50-51)

4. Invest in an identification bracelet

Don't take any chances with your loved one's safety. The episode with the police would have been very different – and certainly easier for everyone had she been wearing an identification bracelet. (Summer 1989 pp. 38-40)

5. Understand that dementia is unpredictable

I learned about the inconsistency of dementia. I was so grateful for the analogy of the tray of light bulbs that one doctor gave me. That explained how Mom would make connections at times and not at other times. It helped me make sense out of the things that didn't make sense. (July 1991 pp. 57-58)

6. Access all the resources you can

Fortunately there are many more resources available today than when I needed them. And it's best to search them out early in order to know what is available when you come to the place of needing it.

Check out books, respite care, day care services, length of waiting lists for seniors' homes, government subsidies for home care, in-house social services, Seniors serving Seniors, financial assistance for making your house safe – like putting handrails in the shower and by the toilet.

For excellent medical and practical information, read *The 36-Hour Day* by Nancy L. Mace and Dr. Peter V. Rabins, John Hopkins University Press.

On-line resources are also available:

http://www.alzheimertoronto.org

This website has a wealth of information and available resources.

http://baycrest.libguides.com/seniorshealthguides

Baycrest's online Seniors Health Resources Page shows resources available in Ontario for loan at no charge. They will send them directly to your home or office along with a postage paid return envelope. Email wellnesslibrary@baycrest.org or call 416-785-2500 x 3374 to request materials.

Wherever you live, your closest Alzheimer Association will be able to direct you to other sources of information and assistance. Again, begin the process of finding resources in the early stages of dementia because once you really need them you may not have the energy to seek them out.

B. Living as the Caregiver

1. Put an alarm on the door before you need it

If you are able to care for someone at home, be sure to have your doors secure. The fact that the present is more and more unfamiliar will drive someone with dementia to find the home of their memory – something that is familiar – and they will do almost anything to get there at any time of the day or night.

Having Mom leave in the middle of the night made us realize if we were to keep her safe and get any sleep ourselves we needed an alarm on the front door which guaranteed I would wake up if she tried to open it. And she did – many times. (Summer 1989 p. 38)

2. Enjoy the humorous in the midst of the difficulties

The experience of one night after we had installed an alarm has given us many a chuckle. I bolted downstairs at the sound of the alarm to find Mom standing at the door still in her pajamas with her purse over her arm. Thinking how cold it was, I simply said, "Oh Mom, you can't go out dressed like that!" She carefully examined herself looking down at her pajamas and declared indignantly, "Why not, they're a matched pair!!" You just have to laugh!

3. Stop to think who you are doing something for

When we brought Mom home to visit after moving to the nursing home, the only thing that made the house seem familiar to her were the paintings on the walls – her own paintings – that sparked some sense of recognition. It became more and more difficult to bring her home – not physically as she was still able to manage but the emotional confusion we created for her began to feel like a torment and we decided it was for our benefit not hers that we were doing this. From then on we simply visited her in the nursing home rather than creating unnecessary confusion for her.

4. Anticipate sudden uncharacteristic behaviours

The greatest shock comes when one day they have no idea who you are and react with anger out of genuine fear. Standing in my kitchen one day, Mom lashed out at me saying, "What are you doing in my kitchen!!" and knocking a cup out of my hand. She was as shocked at her uncharacteristic behavior as I was.

5. Rethink the consequences of any surgery

After our experience would I recommend surgery? Perhaps not. I would certainly ask more questions about the long term benefits and the unexpected consequences.

We thought cataract surgery would improve her ability to enjoy reading and television, and it did once the healing took place. But she couldn't remember why she had a bandage on her eye. I had a wonderful cadre of volunteers from church who sat around the clock with her to keep her from pulling the bandage off, spelling me off. With their help, the results were positive. (October 1992 – January 1993 pp. 60-63)

I don't know what I would do again about a broken hip. Mom never walked after the first break because she couldn't understand the need for pushing through the pain to bring mobility. So it wouldn't have been any different if we had just let the hip heal without the trauma of the hospital visit and the fracture clinic which entailed having to go by wheelchair taxi. I'll never forget the utter panic she experienced as we tried to push her chair into the taxi while she braced herself against the sides of the door with more strength than I knew she had.

A simple remedy would have been to back her in – but who knew!!

The most awful experience for me and it must have been unbelievable for her was trying to hold her down on the table for them to X-ray her hip. Remembering her cries of physical pain mingled with the emotional pain of screaming, "Why are you doing this to me!! You're supposed to be helping me!!" still brings tears. (Summer 1997 – February 1998 p. 66)

6. Enter into their world

I learned that it's smarter to enter into a person's memory world with them than trying to bring them back to my world. I wish someone had told me not to waste my energy trying to keep Mom sorted out. I learned that sharing her memory world – her childhood world – with her was far more comforting to her than all my efforts to help her understand current reality. Once I learned that, we were both less frustrated and I wasn't using up energy uselessly.

And her dreams became more real than reality. Occasionally she would waken and be certain that the person she dreamed of had actually been in her room. It didn't help to contradict her – so I learned to make some excuse for why they hadn't stayed to visit which is what she wanted.

Life was so much better for both of us when I listened to her feelings, reassured her she was loved, gave her a hug and distracted her with something. (April 29 1989 pp. 35-36)

When she shared the enthusiasm of the big house where all the family could stay, and the hope of the farm being cleared by Spring, she was living a wonderful fantasy – why spoil it!! So I simply enthused with her and left her a happy woman. (Preface p. 2; January 1996 pp. 64-65)

7. Recognize that loss of memory means the loss of a sense of time

I learned that leaving Mom for 5 minutes was no different to her than leaving her for 5 days. That significantly lessened the concern I had about taking a vacation. It also took away the pressure of feeling that I needed to be always with her when I was home – something I couldn't do – especially as she would frequently leave whoever was present to her and retreat to her room. (June 1989 p. 38)

C. Caring for Yourself

1. Remember that forgetting things is not the same as dementia

I learned the difference between normal forgetfulness and dementia. Besides the analogy of the tray of light bulbs, the doctor had also given me the analogy of our brain being like a filing drawer full of files. As we get older there are more things filed so it takes longer to find something. That's normal. A person with dementia, however, could search forever and never find it, because it didn't get into the filing drawer in the first place. A person with normal forgetfulness will remember they put the potatoes on to cook when they smell them burning, but someone with dementia will not know they had done so. That information continues to be a comfort to me – almost daily!! (July 1991 pp. 57-58)

2. Be prepared to lose the person piece by piece

I found myself grieving Mom little by little. I lost her in pieces. I lost her as a friend when she could no longer be present to me, as a teacher when she could no longer make sense out of what she was seeing and hearing, as an artist when she could no longer remember how to paint, as a kind and gracious person when she wrote hateful letters out of her paranoia, as a mother when I became her mother, as a grandmother who was always so interested in all her grandchildren when she no longer knew who they were, as a gentle woman when she shocked me with her sudden angry outbursts. Each of those losses was another wave of grief – so much so that I thought I had done all my grieving before she passed away. How surprised I was, then, to discover how huge the hole was that she left in my life and heart.

I learned that grieving little losses along the way doesn't eliminate the pain of the final loss but it's still important to allow yourself to grieve each aspect of the person that disappears. It may be the humour, or the memories, or the companionship, or the comfortable relationship, or the capabilities that are gone. Your relationship will change – perhaps the person changes from being your spouse or parent to become your child. My mother would ask me, when I would take in some clothes for her to try on, "How did you learn to be such a good Mama?" And then when we stood side by side and looked in the mirror, "Why do you have black hair and mine is grey? It should be the other way around?" In her mind, I had clearly become the mother and she the child. (Preface p. 2; Later Reflection p. 18; Eulogy pp. 68-72)

3. Find support for yourself as well as the one you care for

I learned that sometimes it is not the person with dementia who needs the strongest support or greatest ministry. It may be you.

I have learned to let myself be ministered to. Independence is not a Christian value – it is our society's value. Interdependence is Biblical. And we need to learn how to receive the ministry of other people.

Draw your community around you and help them to understand how they can be a source of encouragement to both the one suffering the debilitating and fearful consequences of dementia, and you as the individual or family caring for that person.

What I wished for but didn't have the energy to ask for was someone to do the government paper work for the income tax deductions for our hired caregiver. I was required to file reports of CPP, OHIP, and Income Tax deductions every month as if I were running a business. Computer glitches with the forms were common and getting through to a person was sometimes impossible. I finally got attention by addressing a letter "To the Computer"!!

Let others relieve you of anything they can to minimize the constant drain on your energy.

4. Learn how to grieve well

Change is not always bad, but any change brings loss – and that requires grieving. Only when you have grieved the loss of the old can you embrace the new reality. That was a hard lesson to learn as I did not want to embrace many of the new realities and especially not the reality that my mother felt abandoned by family.

5. Know that encouragement requires truth and compassion

As we spend time with people who need encouragement, their constant questions push us to seek truth. If we remember that God is the source of truth and the source of our compassion, we will not be as easily overwhelmed.

One significant truth is that disease and death are a part of this life and there are things to be talked about. If this life is lived from a temporal perspective, death is a tragedy, but if lived from an eternal perspective, death is both an end to be grieved and a beginning to be celebrated. It's really just another change.

These are some truths that have helped me embrace life's realities:

- grieving and gratitude are not mutually exclusive
- joy and pain can co-exist
- we are not able to fully understand the mysteries of life and death
- I need to grieve
- I can't always have answers
- God does not promise us freedom from pain and suffering
- we do NOT understand the full impact of sin and its consequences in this world
- we live in a fallen world and that brings pain
- God gives us a community to be supportive
- God understands the mixture of emotions

- pain is not punishment for sin but a gift of God to let us know something is wrong
- value does not depend on usefulness
- God is big enough for anything life brings

I learned that it is <u>not</u> true that:

- because someone's fear is not rational, it is not real
- pain must be avoided at all cost
- I have no right to grieve because my grief cannot be as bad as yours
- your experience of any event is the same as my experience
- truth will be devastating

I learned to reject the things people say that are not helpful. It's not helpful to:

- tell people what they already know, i.e. "You need to get help"
- tell them what they should do or should have done
- assume that today's feelings are permanent
- say, "I know exactly how you feel." They d<u>on't</u> – they c<u>an't</u>
- explain God's action; i.e. God is testing your faith, etc.
- explain anything
- ask and then not listen
- avoid the topic
- avoid the person
- focus on self – "At least you have your mother. I lost mine!"
- assume your values are shared: "Just put her in a home!"

I learned that truth with compassion acknowledges that:

- being lost is frightening
- the future may be too fearful to face – that getting through one day is enough at the moment
- when reality doesn't match our expectations, we need time to adjust to reality

- we have the right to feel whatever we are feeling even if others don't think we should
- it's good to ask the questions even when you know there are no answers
- it is not necessary to have answers – but it is necessary to allow people to verbalize the questions
- pat answers don't suffice

And I learned that it <u>is</u> helpful for caregivers to have someone who will:

- allow time to process new information and new experiences
- allow space for healing
- ask how you're feeling rather than assuming
- really LISTEN!
- acknowledge the reality, <u>and</u> the emotions
- focus on you and your current needs rather than themselves
- find out what support looks like at the moment
- alleviate responsibilities – do something FOR you
- offer what they are able to give – be specific

To the extent that I was able to balance truth with compassion, I was able to minister to Mom – give encouragement to face another day or perhaps even just another brief minute – to face her fears with courage and experience some joy.

To the extent that others were able to open my eyes to truth and touch my heart with compassion, they ministered to me – allowing me to face my fears with courage and experience some joy.

6. Take time to be still with God

The place of understanding is in the presence of God. David experienced this and speaks of it in Psalm 73:

> *When I tried to understand all this, it was oppressive to me 'til I entered the sanctuary of God; then I understood.*

David is speaking of a specific situation, but I think the truth is applicable to all situations. We try to understand but cannot with our own striving. Understanding, or truth, comes when we allow ourselves to be in the sanctuary – that quiet place of peace – with God.

Postscript - 2014

All of this seems like a dream now. The good memories predominate. The sadness has lost its edge.

Mom didn't continue to paint. She started out really well – and then kept going over and over the same area until she made it all muddy which of course upset her as she knew it didn't look right. But it was certainly worth the try.

And where's Fred? Fred's not here anymore either.

We said it so often that it became the family joke. I even took this picture of a restaurant in downtown Toronto.

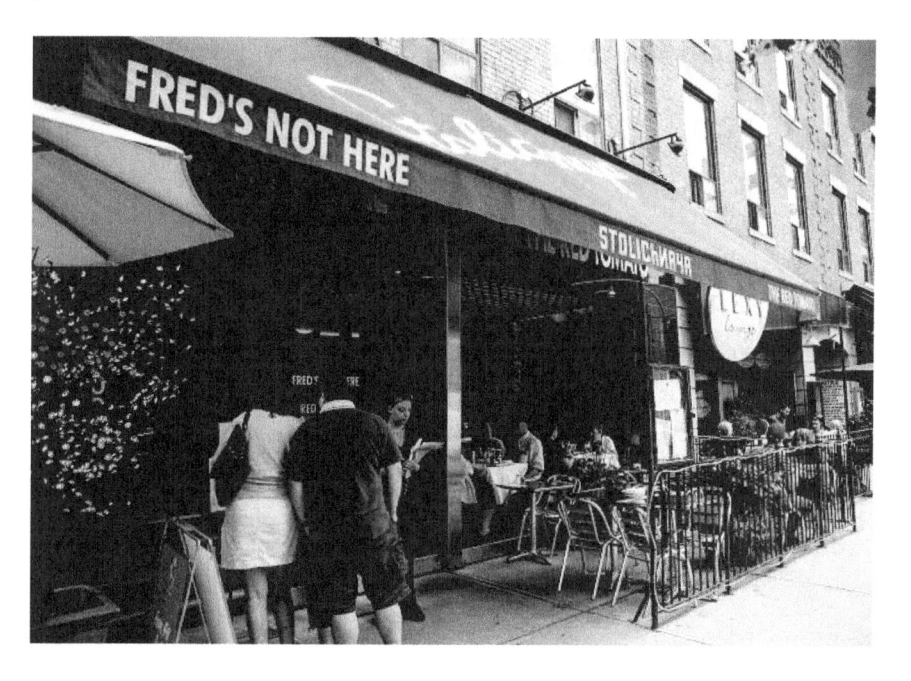

When Dad died, his body was sent to a larger centre for cremation. When his ashes arrived back at the funeral home, the funeral director called my sister, Gayle, with the message, "Fred's here!!" and was, I'm sure, quite startled by her reaction. She simply couldn't stifle her laughter!

In Dad's last few years his agnostic stance changed to belief and so he is with Mom and she no longer has to ask, "Where's Fred?" or to hear the words, "Fred's not here." They are finally home together again.

> Lynn,
>
> Please take me home - That is "take me to Fred's place (that is mine also)" I need to have someone to talk to, not to scold me as that seems to be all anyone <u>does.</u>
>
> Take me to my Dad's home up on the Hill.
>
> Please ---F.A. <u>thanks</u>

Appendix

A further sampling of Mom's notes – her valiant attempt to make sense out of her utter confusion.

> Frances Adcock –
> What happened to everybody – I have been alone and wonder what happened & why. –
> I need to know what & where I go from here. –

Dear Family
There is no one left but me - I am in a room alone - I can hear movements and talking in other places (the hall and stairway) but no one to talk to - <u>I would like to go home</u> in the morning please - <u>come and get me</u> and tell me <u>how</u> to get home. Love M.F.

Tell <u>John</u> and <u>Ruth</u> as well as <u>Gayle</u> and <u>Gerry</u> where we are and please find us - and "tell us" where we are and what we should "do" or "go" pdq
I am all alone now except for the TV

Love as ever, Mom

Today I feel sad and so alone. I would love to have been able to visit while Fred was buzzing about. It is sad to be alone when I would have loved to have had a family visit -----It feels as tho' all I have done or have spent my life at, was to pay bills and worry about how long the money would last. Now I am alone at Lynn's. She is out teaching and I'm just putting in time, and need some suggestions. Roger had a stint at the hospital but is doing fine now. They have a gal doing the housework and meals which I enjoy after all these years. However I would like to have gone visiting with Fred to see the family.

Dear Lynn,
I do not understand this letter to Lynn from Fred, do you?
I am still me and worry about family - I need them all.
I have given help to all and any of the family as they needed it" and now I am left alone and find it hard to understand - I have always had family until now, why?
    I won't worry but I wonder what he is talking about etc
Love Mom A.

Dear Lynn - I came in one door and you went out the other. I visited for a while but you didn't come back so I stayed until late - will have to go.
Love Mom A

Dear Ruth and John and any others
   Why don't you come to visit me.
I need my friends now as always. I am so lonesome, I wonder why —
   I need family and friends, why do I never see any of my family anymore — (I miss my Dad and the rest of the family) — I am alone tonight and can't understand — I have always had family and friends and wonder where they are. I need to find them as I have always had lots of friends and can't understand. I need all of them — please help me —

NEVER IN MY LIFE HAVE I BEEN LEFT WITHOUT REASON AND WARNING so it is hard to understand — Mom

Don't leave me here alone — please — Frances

Don't forget
I'm upstairs and
alone =
           M. F. Q.
I need to go home.

It would have been nice if Fred had given me a trip around to see the family. I would have loved that but I am no good to get going on my own especially to find my way about.

> I need to know
> ① Why am I here
> ② family do not come.
> ③ I need to have company old friends & family.
> ④ I need to help in any way I can.
> — Frances
> & Mom

Is there a bus that will take me home? I do need help and advice as to how to get home - soon -   The picture of my family must have come from a friend or relative. Do tell me about it - also about the bus that picks up from here.
Thank you, whoever

Lynn - there is something really wrong - I have never been give a job or a time to do anything - I need some responsibility to work or talk or ???   Just being a "nothing" human is <u>not good</u> for me or anyone - why me

> I thought I would get out of the way by going to bed + not disturbing any one but I have been alone for 2 hours and not a soul to talk to — for me, that is a sad state of affairs — I need company some one to talk
> I feel so alone and ~~sad~~

I'd like to know where I am - or should "go" or "be" - now!! I need to know about a lot of things "here and now" etc. Please give me some information about you and where I should be - I am one who likes everyone and every place but I need a "name" for it and also some references as to "need" for a place - where I am needed.

I do not know what to expect of tomorrow - each day hands out a different bit of news - so I will expect whatever comes. I need to rest now - perhaps tomorrow will shed some new light on my life.
But for just now - good night - with love, Frances

Hi to the Family (where are they)
I need your advice again. Come in and tell me about myself and (what else)

I will not be staying here – it is so lonely and dreary. I can come and get my clothes someday soon – there are places and other ways of getting educated. I will try them. It is more lonely here than on the farm. The animals there will talk to anyone. I will come and talk to you some day again. It is bedtime now – as ever Frances Adcock

To John
I need your help. What happened last night? Where's Fred? Did he leave and why am I here? Where has the family gone? Please help me to find them.
Love Mom – I feel so lost.

I don't want to live alone – I need someone to talk to & who will also talk & explain to me –

Dear Fred and Family

Why am I here and alone? I have wandered around trying to find family – so just gave up.

Why did you do this to me? I am sick and do not believe I deserved such treatment but now what should I believe.

I'm tired and sick and alone. Mom A

There is nothing as sad as growing OLD.
I said "OLD", not OLDer, just OLD..
I have enjoyed my life –
    even to getting older and wiser?
But now tho I'm older & should be wiser
I feel sad and lonely –
Why am I alone?
Where is Fred?
Is he getting older or wiser?
Why doesn't he write?

Dear Lynn

What am I supposed to do? Do I act? I really have feelings. How do I control them and me? I need to talk. I feel as if I am in a thick cloud and can't see my way out.

Love Mom

Dear Dad, —
    I really need to get out. I always like to hear the birds and to listen to see the little ~~anima~~ animals crawling & hunting about. And spring is the best time for all living creatures to move about even me. I do need to get out, I am lost. Please rescue me, I need to go home. Do come soon.

    Please come in and wake me — I need someone to talk to — Why am I here and where should I be?
    This seems like home but please let me know.
        Love
          Mom.

Dear John, —

I feel so alone tonight and wonder what I should do — Could I go to be with my family — I am so alone — no one cares that I am alone or need company — I am sure there are "homes" where I can help little ones to read and draw; please try to find one.

I have helped beginners read and draw and "sing" — I would like to do that again.

Please find a home for me where they want me to help.

Love
mom

Lynn - why - (get the police if worried)

Please help. I <u>need</u> your help now - to know what, why and where I should go. Please explain "to help" why where and when - (I need to know) - so do you.

Love Mom F

 I don't want to get sick and right now I feel it. Where is Fred? Why am I lost? and alone? Please "explain" -
If Fred is happy then I will not worry - but let me know. Fred will have to tell me what and why - and tell me what to expect and do.

About the Author

Lynn has written two books prior to this one. *Gender or Giftedness: A challenge to rethink the basis for leadership within the Christian community* was a response to the questions posed to her by students about the role of women when she served Tyndale University College and Seminary in Toronto, Canada, as Dean of Students and Vice President of Student Development. This book has been translated into German, French, Arabic and Croatian.

Her second book, *Mentoring: Leaving Legacy,* grew out of her personal involvement with women of all ages who sought her out as an encourager on their personal journey and the request of participants in a weekend leadership conference in Germany to have her teaching notes available for them in book form. It was published first in Germany.

As a representative of the Evangelical Fellowship of Canada to the World Evangelical Alliance, Lynn connected with many International women which led to her invitations to teach in various countries on the topics of gender, leadership and mentoring.

Lynn is one of the founders of NextLEVEL Leadership, an international organization devoted to encouraging Christian women to develop the character, competence and confidence necessary to have a credible voice in their spheres of influence in ministry, profession or the marketplace.

When she brought her mother who was suffering from dementia to live with her, she found journalling helped to release her own stress and keep her family informed. As she observed close friends and family members facing the same care-giving role, she decided to share her journey. Much progress has been made since her experience – in terms of understanding dementia and the support available – but the emotional journey is still difficult and she believes that caregivers need a special kind of courage.

Lynn and her husband Roger enjoy spending time with their adult children and grandchildren as well as opportunities for travel, teaching, mentoring and a variety of church and community activities.